Thriving in Non-Monogamy
An Ethical Slut's Guide

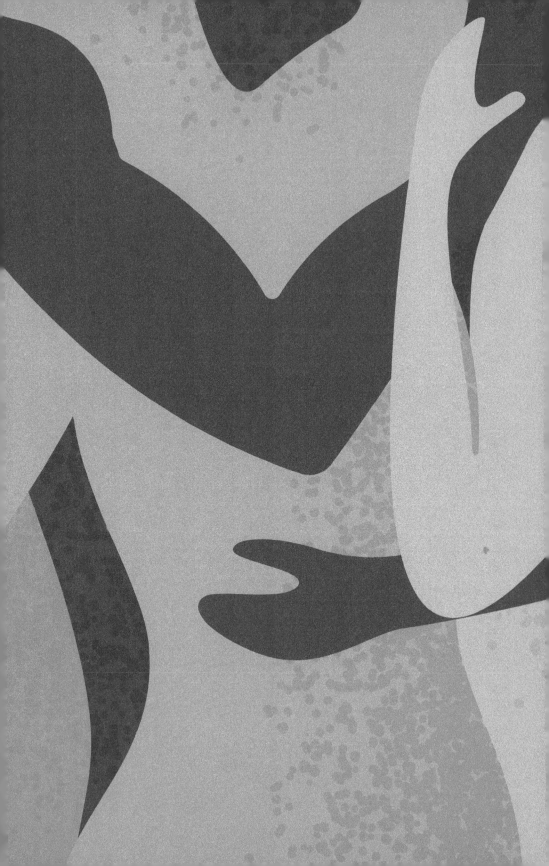

Thriving in Non-Monogamy

An Ethical Slut's Guide

Overcome Jealousy, Enjoy Sex, and Honor Yourself

Erin Davidson, RCC, MA

ROCKRIDGE
PRESS

Interior and Cover Designer: Erik Jacobsen
Art Producer: Sara Feinstein
Editor: Brian Sweeting
Production Manager: Riley Hoffman
Production Editor: Sigi Nacson

Illustrations used under license from Shutterstock.com
Author photo courtesy of Amy Davidson

ISBN: Print 978-1-64739-621-3 | Ebook 978-1-64739-622-0
R1

This book is dedicated to my clients.

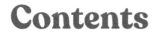

Contents

Introduction

We are all deserving and capable of enjoying fulfilling romantic and sexual relationships. Connection is the key to living a full life. Connection to yourself first and foremost—awareness of your emotions, body sensations, values, and needs. Believing fully in your inherent worth, flaws and all. Connecting to others through empathy, vulnerability, and reliability. We live in a culture of dichotomies: mind vs. body, masculine vs. feminine, monogamy vs. non-monogamy. Often our work is not to learn, but to unlearn, to look at the messaging we've been fed from society and decide what works for us and what doesn't, and then to come back to the wisdom within.

This book is divided into three parts: part I asks if ethical non-monogamy (ENM) is right for you, part II guides the process of opening your relationship, and part III addresses common challenges and how to thrive in spite of them. Non-monogamy is a broad topic that can vary significantly by culture. In this book, when I say, "in our society/culture," I am referring to a North American context. Throughout the book you'll find key words and terms in bold, with definitions in the Glossary (see page 172).

I am a sex therapist and writer. I am a firm believer in the healing power of pleasure and being kinder to ourselves. I am also a therapy nerd. I think society at large benefits when we take the time to better understand ourselves in all our messiness. Because of this, I will frequently reference therapy as a modality for healing. I want to acknowledge that healing takes multiple forms, and only you can know what the right path is for you.

Throughout the book you'll follow the stories of people from a variety of genders, sexual orientations, and relationship structures. These are not real people; they are representations of the many diverse clients who have shared their experiences with me. This is to protect the confidentiality of my clients, as well as to capture a wider range of experiences.

The purpose of this book is to help you reflect on what your ideal relationship structure is. This process opens up many questions that challenge our society's typical ways of thinking about relationships. If something resonates, I encourage you to dive deeper. This book is a jumping-off point. It isn't the whole story or the only way of doing things. Glean what works for you and leave the rest. There are as many ways of being in a relationship as there are relationships in this world.

*   *   *

When you're a sex therapist, one of the many (*many*) questions people ask you at parties is "Why?"

If I could talk to my teenage self, she would be shocked to know my chosen career. I grew up in a **sex-negative** environment. From a young age, I internalized the rules of being a "good girl," not the least of which demanded no sex before marriage. As I got older—and I moved away for school, studied psychology, fell in love, had sex—I started to untangle the messages I had been force-fed about sexuality and relationships.

The Venn diagram of sex and shame became one big circle when I was sexually assaulted in my early 20s. As most survivors do, I fully blamed myself. I was in crisis, feeling that the realm of sexuality had caused me nothing but pain. I remember saying to my therapist, "I just wish sex wasn't a thing."

As a part of my healing process, I sought out all the books, podcasts, and courses I could find on sexuality. I started to understand the harmful systems in our culture that perpetuate sexual violence against women and particularly women of color. I began to find empowerment through using my voice. I wrote online about my assault and pursued a master's degree in counseling where I interviewed sexual assault survivors for my thesis. I started to learn that pleasure is healing—be it through food, or rest, or orgasms—and that I was worthy of feeling all the beautiful sensations my body was capable of. I realized I wanted to train to be a sex therapist to help others emancipate themselves from shame. I hope this book helps you on your own journey of learning and unlearning—to create a life on your own terms.

PART I

Is Non-Monogamy Right For You?

Whether you have arrived at this book from a point of curiosity or a desire to enhance an existing understanding, I have no doubt that immersing yourself in this material will deepen how you practice relationships. As a sex therapist, **ethical non-monogamy (ENM)** is one of my favorite topics to discuss with my clients because it encourages people to consider a path separate from the typical age-associated relationship milestones, sometimes referred to as the relationship escalator. There is no one-size-fits-all approach to sex and relationships, and my goal is not to pit ENM against monogamy or to argue one style as superior. Instead, I hope the material can serve as a catalyst for you to break down your own personal relationship expectations to rebuild in a way that works best for you.

We'll start by examining different arrangements of non-monogamous relationships and the role of sex in ENM, and finish with a self-assessment of needs and fears when living as an **ethical slut**. Sex and relationships can be powerful and transformative forces in our lives. The relationship structure that is the best fit for each of us varies from person to person and can change throughout our lives. This section is designed to help you consider the different arrangements of ethical non-monogamy and whether there are pieces that might fit in your relationship right now.

Recognizing Your Relationship Values

Carving out space to clarify your relationship values is a vital step in building a life of fulfilling connection. Your values mirror what is most meaningful to you: the type of person you want to be, your purpose for being in a relationship, and how others think of you. When you are clear on your relationship values, they can serve as direction and motivation to guide the choices you make.

All worthwhile relationships go through challenges and take work, whether they are monogamous or polyamorous arrangements. An ENM relationship may offer you transformative experiences that you never could have imagined and still have points within that same relationship when you are so anxious that all you eat are animal crackers for 24 hours. Polyamorous relationships require more effort, simply because all relationships take effort and when you introduce more people, more relational dynamics need to be considered and communicated. During the challenging times, what I have consistently heard from my ENM clients is that coming back to their values keeps them grounded in their relational choices. To assist you in determining what your own values are, the following chapter will be as much a discussion of positive relationship values as of relationship arrangements.

What Is an Ethical Slut?

If you've heard the term "ethical slut," it's likely that you've read Dossie Easton and Janet Hardy's book of the same name. If you're not familiar, a person of any gender can claim the term "ethical slut," per Easton and Hardy, if they "have courage to lead life according to the radical proposition that sex is nice and pleasure is good for you." *The Ethical Slut* was first published in 1997 and was considered to be somewhat of a bible for budding polyamorists. However, this call to radically celebrate sex with many partners may inadvertently send the message that polyamory is only about sex.

Sexual desire is powerful and important, and many people do begin to explore ENM because they want to explore their sexuality with someone new. Yet, to reduce living as an ethical slut to only sex is to miss what is at the heart of ENM, which is intimacy and relationships. In short: ethical non-monogamy is about more than sex, but sex is important.

In the more than two decades since the first edition of *The Ethical Slut*, much of what was written is no longer such a radical notion, especially for younger generations. A lot of the early work of books on non-monogamy was to help people untangle their traditional views of monogamy—to question them, understand where they come from—in a sense to "undo" monogamy before being able to understand a different way of being in relationship with others. This is not the same way many folks born after 1980 now approach relationships; for a lot of younger people, non-monogamy is in the zeitgeist, and open relationships are now frequently portrayed in music, movies, and TV. A recent poll of US adults showed that 43 percent of millennials view non-monogamy as their ideal relationship option.

Although visibility and understanding of ENM is becoming more commonplace, it is certainly still a dramatic diversion from the social norm. To add to this, many of us may intellectually agree that "sex is nice and pleasure is good for you," but as a result of growing up in a society with a long history of capitalistic, patriarchal, puritan messaging, we still have a lot of **sex-negativity** to untangle. The messaging we receive about sex can really mess with your mind.

Sex is both glorified and thrust into the shadows at the same time. We are bombarded with sex on our magazine covers, Instagram feeds, and Internet searches. Yet, the number of sexual partners someone has had is usually grounds for judgment, women's bodies and clothing choices are policed, and talking about sex in most circumstances is considered taboo. And for marginalized groups, namely those who are non-white, fat-bodied, differently-abled, or in the LGBTQ+ community, expressing sexuality and claiming pleasure publicly is revolutionary. I am firmly aligned with Easton and Hardy when I state, Sex is transformative and pleasure is healing.

Sex is transformative and pleasure is healing.

What Is "Ethical"?

Let's break things down. To be ethical in the context of relationships means that you act in a way that values the importance of free will, and you aim to make the other person feel loved, cared for, and secure. To do this requires practicing and developing emotional literacy and communication skills. This behavior includes the understanding that it is your responsibility to do the work of figuring out your own needs, expressing them, communicating your boundaries, and practicing effective and clear communication through disagreements.

To be ethical in a relationship involves honesty and integrity. This means honoring any relationship agreements, whether they be safer sex practices or expectations of monogamy. Relationally focused honesty, however, is not a free pass for unbridled self-expression. It means being transparent about things that are helpful for the other person to know and that affect the relationship dynamic. For example, telling a partner that your ex gave better head than they do is probably *not* something that currently impacts the relationship or is helpful for them to know. However, let's say that you had unprotected sex with a new partner and have not yet been tested; this is something that might not be a pleasant piece of information, but it is vital to disclose because it does affect the relationship.

With regard to being ethical in sexual relationships, I find it helpful to default to Dan Savage's **campsite rule**. He wrote this rule to specifically apply to an older person starting a relationship with someone significantly younger, but I find it fits well for sex in general. The premise is that you should leave your sexual partner better, or at least as good, physically and emotionally, as you found them. This refers to decisions about contraception, STIs (sexually transmitted infections), sense of safety, and well-being.

Acting ethically in a relationship is a key component for trust to develop. It may be surprising to hear that trust isn't something that just happens in relationships. When someone says, "Trust me," it is actually a ridiculous request. Trust doesn't happen on demand; it occurs when people show up consistently and act with integrity. It is not possible to trust without also balancing risk. When we trust someone, we are deciding that they have shown up for us reliably enough that we consider them to be worth the risk of getting hurt. Take, for example, the classic "trust fall" exercise. The person chooses to trust by falling backward, and in so doing, they are actually taking the risk that they will be dropped.

> *Trust doesn't happen on demand; it occurs when people show up consistently and act with integrity.*

In ethical relationships, we are choosing to take the risk of trusting another person. We choose to hold the other person in goodwill and trust they will do the same for us. All relationships end, whether through breakup or death, so when we enter into close relationships with others, we make the decision that the risk of getting hurt by opening ourselves and being vulnerable with one another is worth the deep connections it allows.

Values and Ideals

A big part of deciding what relationship structure works best for you is by seeing whether it aligns with your relationship values and ideals. As I mentioned earlier, being clear on your relationship values can also help you keep perspective about what is important to you and stay the

RECLAIMING SLUTS

For many, the word "slut" holds a stinging negative connotation. It certainly has been used historically to cut down women. It may be confusing to see this word spoken as a compliment or worn as a badge of honor. The meaning behind the word "slut" has changed over the years, but some of the most common understandings now include "a woman who has many sexual partners." When this definition is more closely examined, it is no wonder there have been movements to reclaim the term. This definition is only an insult if you view women or sex negatively. Because you've arrived at this book, I'm going to imagine that you at least dabble in sex-positivity and feminism, and from that perspective, why wouldn't being a person who has frequent sex be celebrated?

course during the more challenging times in your relationships. How exactly, then, do you figure out your relationship values? In addition to the values of honesty, integrity, and trust discussed previously, some other common relationship values include freedom, self-awareness, positivity, and fun.

Many of my clients have said that the mutual valuing of freedom can be one of the most powerful components of ethically non-monogamous relationships, because they know that their partner is with them because they want to be, rather than from any sense of obligation. Valuing self-awareness can look like appreciating a partner who demonstrates an understanding of their strengths and weaknesses, as well as the ability to express their emotions and apologize for their mistakes. It can also look like a commitment to personal growth through taking on new challenges, going to therapy, or attending support meetings.

A partner who is able to hold a positive attitude and find the fun in life can be valuable to many people. Positivity can come in the form of an optimistic outlook on life, and it can also show up in the way someone communicates. When partners value speaking kindly to one another, providing mutual support, and saying nice things to each other, it can dramatically impact the level of satisfaction in the relationship. Sometimes we seek relationships with particular people because they simply make things more fun. We also sometimes gravitate toward relationships with people who are strong in the areas where we struggle. For people who tend to experience a higher rate of anxiety and worry, they may particularly value a partner who can help them see the lighter side of life.

To figure out your own values, it can be helpful to reflect on your most positive experience in a relationship and your most negative. It may also be helpful to journal a paragraph on each experience and pick out what qualities were present each time. What did trust look like? How did you speak to each other? Were any topics off-limits? What was your monogamy arrangement? Both positive and negative relationship experiences can be great clues to what is important to you and what your ideal relationship looks like.

What Is an *Unethical* Slut?

When someone moves through relationships with a lack of self-understanding or connection to a deeper value system, it is easy for them to cause harm. **Unethical sluthood** includes any action that controls, limits, or disregards the well-being of others. This behavior would also fall into a category of emotional abuse. Other forms of emotional abuse include criticizing, gaslighting, withholding affection, and using threats.

When someone is trapped in an emotionally abusive relationship, it is often challenging for them to realize it. This is because the attempts made by the abuser to exert power and control often start small and build over time, like the temperature dial slowly being turned up in a room until it is unbearable. It is also confusing because behaviors like gaslighting are used to disempower by distorting someone's understanding of reality. When abuse comes from someone we love, we are left to grapple with how this same person would also want to hurt us. If you think you might be in an abusive relationship, the non-profit organization RAINN (the Rape, Abuse & Incest National Network) is available for 24-hour support.

Unethical sexual behavior is at best selfish and at worst coercive and destructive. It may look like disregarding other people's sexual health by never getting tested, hiding one's STI (sexually transmitted infection) status, or removing a condom covertly during sex (a literal "dick" move called *stealthing*). It can look like treating a sexual partner as an object rather than a person or seeking sex as a conquest or prize. This type of behavior is often seen in **hookup culture** on university campuses, where there is pressure for people to seek sex for prestige or a reputation boost, rather than for connection with another human being.

Another unfortunately common example includes when an otherwise monogamous couple wants to add in a **third** for a one-off sexual experience. Sometimes couples can see this third person as existing solely to meet the couple's sexual needs and forget that this third person is also an individual with their own desires and dislikes. Finally, being an unethical slut can also include stepping outside the agreements in the relationship and cheating on a partner.

Ethical Non-Monogamy vs. Cheating

It is a misconception that it is not possible to cheat in an ethically non-monogamous relationship. In ENM relationships, it is common to have a relatively formalized agreement that outlines what behaviors are and are not acceptable, what the boundaries of openness are, as well as the amount of disclosure that is expected within the partnership about other relationships. Cheating in a monogamous or non-monogamous relationship means stepping outside the agreed-upon boundaries. For example, if a non-monogamous couple has a rule that all sex outside their relationship should be safer sex, and one partner is not using a condom with their other partners, this would be stepping outside the relationship.

Monogamous relationships have these agreements as well; however, they are often never explicitly discussed because many people simply look to the prevailing societal expectations. This can often cause trouble in relationships. Particularly in our ever-evolving technological landscape, it becomes more and more difficult to classify cheating. Is it cheating to flirt through DMs? Or to masturbate to photos of an ex? Or to chat with a cam girl? Many monogamous couples have never talked about their relationship boundaries and limits together.

Because ethical non-monogamy steps outside the societal expectation and norms, being in an ENM relationship often means designing the relationship parameters from scratch and pulling on more limited relationship models, which may not always fit their individual relationship/s. This means partners in ENM relationships will typically have more negotiations together about their relationship structure. It is important to remember, however, that the expectations of monogamy are also complicated and certainly do not work well for everyone. People in monogamous relationships very much benefit from taking the time to discuss their own personalized limits and boundaries. Later on, in chapter 4, there will be space for you to reflect on identifying and setting your own boundaries and establishing relationship agreements.

Non-Monogamy, Polyamory, and Open Relationships

At first glance, polyamory, non-monogamy, and open relationships may seem like they can be used interchangeably. It is true that some of these terms can overlap, but there are also significant differences. Non-monogamy is considered to be the umbrella term under which polyamory and open relationships fall. **Polyamory** is a subset of ethical non-monogamy because all parties involved are aware of and consent to the arrangement of being in a relationship with others with the possibility of falling in love. An **open relationship** is also a non-monogamous formation in which two people who are already in a relationship agree that they are free to take new partners. Both open and polyamorous relationships engage in non-monogamy. However, it is possible for people who are non-monogamous to be single, and single folks would not be in an open or polyamorous relationship. Are you with me? Don't worry, it will become clearer in this next section.

Another common misunderstanding is that people sometimes confuse polyamory with the term "polygamy," which refers specifically to a man who has many wives. It is also important to mention that many polyamorous people consider polyamory to be an identity rather than a practice; for example, "Alex is polyamorous" rather than "Alex practices polyamory." This is in contrast to **swingers** (couples who agree to have sex with other couples), who typically consider non-monogamy something that they do through "swinging."

A study conducted with US Census–based quota samples of single adults found that more than one in five American adults reported practicing consensual non-monogamy at some point during their lives. The same proportion was shown regardless of race, religion, age, income, education level, or political affiliation. It was shown, however, that higher rates of men (compared with women) and people with lesbian, gay, or bisexual identities (compared with heterosexual identities) reported engaging in consensual non-monogamy at some point in their lives.

Non-Monogamy

"Non-monogamy" is the broadest term of the bunch, with both polyamory and open relationships considered to be a type of non-monogamy. To be non-monogamous simply means for someone to be involved in more than one sexual or intimate relationship at the same time. A person can identify as non-monogamous and also be single because non-monogamy can also refer to an ideology and identity. This can also be the case with people who are single and still identify as polyamorous.

The practice of non-monogamy can be consensual or non-consensual. Openly dating a variety of people can be a frequent experience of consensual non-monogamy, even for those who go on to be in a monogamous relationship. Non-consensual non-monogamy can vary from someone cheating in the context of their monogamous marriage to dating multiple people at the same time and keeping it a secret. **Consensual non-monogamy** is often used interchangeably with ethical non-monogamy. I gravitate toward the term "ethical non-monogamy" because it includes more than just consent; it is also a valuing of freedom and goodwill toward those involved.

Polyamory

Polyamory (or poly) is a form of relationship where it is understood and accepted that people can create multiple sexual, intimate, and romantic connections with others. The word is based on the Greek word *poly*, meaning many, and the Latin word *amor* for love. Although the act of loving more than one person is not new and has existed in organized forms in many cultures before showing up in North America, the term "polyamory" came into existence in the early 1990s. Although the exact source is debated, it is said that the word was created as a way to describe what type of relationship it *is*, rather than what it *is not* (*non*-monogamy).

Polyamorous folks frequently adopt a primary/secondary relationship formation, which means that they hold one or more central relationships, plus other relationships, which are considered peripheral. There are also arrangements that include multiple equal partnerships. These are often described as a *V*, an *N*, or a *W*, in which each point of the letter refers to a person and the line represents the connection between people. A **polycule** is also a term that is meant to visually represent multiple equal partnerships by invoking the image of how the particles in a molecule are connected. It is possible for a polycule to be closed to other relationships separate from the group (**polyfidelitous**) or open. There are also people who practice **solo/poly**, meaning that they live alone and keep their finances separate even if they are dating, in a relationship, or married.

Open Relationships

This form of non-monogamy refers to couples who are open to partners having sex with people outside their relationship. Open relationships center the primary partnership, so committed partnerships, romantic connections, or love bonds outside the primary couple are not a part of the agreement. The simplest way to differentiate open relationships from polyamorous relationships is that open relationships refer exclusively to sex and poly relationships refer to partnerships.

A couple in an open relationship may be looking for sexual experiences together (a threesome or group experiences), or they may be looking to have sexy adventures separately. Couples sometimes have fun looking for potential partners together on dating apps, at bars, or at sex parties, or they also may do this part of the process individually. A couple may invite a third person in for a sexual experience where all parties participate equally, or one partner may enjoy watching their partner with someone new.

Relationship Anarchy and Hierarchies

People in polyamorous relationships may adopt a hierarchical approach where they have a primary/secondary relationship formation. Often, but not always, this arrangement will occur when a couple has been together for a while in a monogamous arrangement and is looking to add other partners to their relationship, or if the primary couple has ties together like marriage, living together, or children. Many people find labels such as "primary" and "secondary" helpful, to create clarity and understanding of the expectations in the relationship.

Many poly people, however, dislike the way the primary/secondary formation creates hierarchies, and they may opt for an arrangement where they have multiple equal partners. This can be described as a polycule or take the form of the *V, N,* or *W* mentioned previously. **Relationship anarchy** is the term for an approach that many polyamorous people take, which means that no specific types of relationships are privileged over others and any relationship choice is acceptable.

OPEN RELATIONSHIPS
REFLECTED IN CULTURE

As society seems to become more open-minded, we have seen an increase of portrayals of open relationships in pop culture. Some musical examples include Britney Spears's "3," in which she sings about a threesome, or Lou Bega and all his Monicas, Ritas, and Tinas in "Mambo No. 5."

Over the past decade, Netflix has served a delightful array of TV series and movies featuring open relationships. Although they aren't always the most accurate or flattering portrayals of non-monogamy, it is encouraging to see more visibility of a variety of relationship styles. Some dysfunctional portrayals include the show *Wanderlust*, where married couple Joy and Alan decide to try to rejuvenate their relationship by opening it up after they both sort of cheat on each other. In *House of Cards*, Claire and Frank show a cold and occasionally predatory approach to extramarital sex. The series *Easy* follows a variety of different character storylines, with one episode showcasing a couple looking to have a threesome and another string of episodes following a married couple navigating the trials of opening up their relationship.

It seems to be the case that the version of open relationships most frequently portrayed in the media is that of the middle-class, white, married, heterosexual couple. The show *She's Gotta Have It*, the TV series reboot of the 1986 Spike Lee film of the same name, follows Nola Darling and her multiple relationships. Although Darling has been criticized for her polyamory being rooted in "selfishness, uncertainty, and narcissism," her presence is still incredibly valuable as a queer Black woman who is radically honest and unapologetic about her own pleasure. In the future, it is important that we see more diversity on screens.

People who hold this perspective strongly value free will for themselves and their partners, spontaneity, and the removal of obligations from relationships. Relationship anarchists also decentralize the romantic couple as the most important relationship and shifts equal value to other forms of relationships, such as friendship. A beautiful example of this decentering of the couple comes from Clementine Morrigan, a polyamorous author who writes about the intersections of trauma, attachment, and polyamory. Morrigan wrote in their zine *Love without Emergency*, "Hetero-monogamous scripts expect people to 'grow out of the roommate phase' and move in with a partner, and although there is nothing wrong with living with your partner, it is not the only possibility for building a loving home or a loving partnership."

A Range of Relationships

We live in a society of **compulsory monogamy**, where monogamy is the unquestioned norm and expectation. Because of this, many people live their lives following a script, blind to the infinite possibilities in which relationships can take shape. As a therapist, I frequently see people suppress and banish what they need and want in relationships because it does not line up with what society expects. We face very real pressure to try to match the monogamous expectations in order to have a societally defined "successful relationship." However, with divorce rates at close to 50 percent, it is clear that compulsory monogamy does not work for everyone.

Our sexual and relational desires are powerful—more powerful than we often realize—and when we suppress these needs, it just gives them more momentum to pop into our lives in unexpected ways. Being honest with your deepest relational and sexual desire can be one of the most important things you do in your life. I'm not saying this is easy; there can be grief in letting go of one vision of yourself to make room for another, or perhaps accepting that you will not fulfill your family's expectations. You may receive more judgment for this arrangement than if you just tried to blend in with the monogamous crowd. Remember, though: It is a fallacy to think there is *one* template that defines a successful relationship. There are as many approaches to relationships as there are people on this planet. The following list is just a sample of some of the limitless potential relationship structures.

Single

Being single is the state of being unattached to a committed relationship. A single person may be dating and looking for a partner, or they may be content solo. A single person may or may not be having sex with others. Because of the compulsory monogamy pressure in our society, single people often face stigma. Ironically, I have observed in my clinical practice that many people look back fondly at the times in their lives when they were single. Efforts have been made to reclaim what it means to be happy and single. Actress Emma Watson popularized the term **self-partnered**.

Asexuality and Celibacy

These terms may seem similar because they both include the decision not to have sex. However, the reasoning behind this decision is vastly different. To be **celibate** is to abstain from sex, often for religious, spiritual, or personal reasons. **Asexuality**, on the other hand, is considered a sexual identity, in which a person experiences little to no sexual attraction. The term is sometimes shortened to **ace** and has also been described to be on a spectrum of experiencing attraction. **Gray-A** refers to falling somewhere along the spectrum of asexuality, with being somewhat sexual; this includes people who feel sexual attraction only after experiencing a romantic or emotional connection with someone (termed **demisexual**).

Platonic Relationships

Platonic relationships refer to a strong relationship connection between two people without engaging sexually with one another. A platonic relationship can also be considered a friendship. These relationships are often based on shared interests, a deep understanding of one another, or similar outlooks on life. Platonic relationships may start from professional or personal connections. A common term of endearment for a platonic relationship between two male-identifying people is a **bromance**. Relationship anarchists often push for equal valuation of platonic relationships as well as romantic and sexual relationships.

Friends with Benefits

Friends with benefits is a sexual arrangement between friends where there is no intention of turning the connection into a more committed relationship. People may be friends with benefits if they are not currently looking for a relationship, or if they believe they would be incompatible in a relationship together. The term **fuckbuddies** is also commonly used synonymously. In the early 2010s, the plot of the fuck-buddies who later fall in love seemed to be quite popular, with films such as *Friends with Benefits* and *No Strings Attached*.

Monogamish

Longtime sex advice columnist Dan Savage coined the term **monogamish** as a description for the type of open relationship he has with his husband. In Savage's marriage, they are mostly monogamous with each other, but allow space for sex outside the relationship. They would be considered each other's primary partners, and the extramarital sex may occur together or separately. They also hold an expectation of honesty if someone has another sexual experience. The term the **new monogamy** has also been used to describe a type of monogamous relationship that allows space for other emotional and sexual connections.

Partnership

A "partner," in the context of relationships, is a person someone is married to or has a romantic or sexual connection with. This term is often preferred to labels such as husband, wife, boyfriend, or girlfriend because it is not gender-specific. The term can also refer to the type of connection where you are associated together through work or play, such as a business, dance, or tennis partner.

Other Arrangements

Casual relationships: A casual relationship, or casual dating, is a relationship that is usually primarily sexual but free of any extra commitments or labels.

Ménage à trois: This refers to a sexual act, rather than a relationship, in which three people engage sexually with one another at the same time.

Swinging: When a primary couple interacts sexually with other primary couples.

Group sex: Also commonly called an *orgy*, when multiple people get together to have sex in various formations.

BDSM/kink: The acronym *BDSM* stands for bondage and discipline, dominance and submission, and sadomasochism. *Kink* is often used as a blanket term that includes BDSM as well as sexual behaviors and identities that are considered non-conventional. People in the BDSM/kink communities can form deep and meaningful relationships through this shared identity. Whereas some engage in BDSM/kink periodically or recreationally (frequently at BDSM *dungeons* or *play parties*), some form 24/7 *D/s* (dominance and submission) relationships.

Polyfidelity: A *polycule* or group of polyamorous people who are closed to outside relationships.

Triad/quad: A group of three or four people, respectively, who are in a consensual non-monogamous relationship together.

Line family: A term used to describe a consensually non-monogamous relationship where people are connected in their romantic and sexual relationship with some but not all the people connected by the formation. Some common formations include a *V*, *N*, and *W*, where each point of the letter indicates a person, and the line is the connection between them.

Metamour: In ethically non-monogamous relationships, this refers to someone's partner's partner.

Kitchen table poly: A description for a polyamorous relationship in which all partners get along well enough that they could sit around a kitchen table and share a cup of coffee together. This typically refers to an amicable relationship with one's **metamour**.

Common Misperceptions of Non-Monogamy

In any situation, going against social expectations can bring unique challenges. Take, for example, the teen who chooses to become a musician after high school rather than pursue a post-secondary degree. This teen will likely face questions and assumptions from others about why they've selected this path and what this lifestyle choice means. People will project their own experiences and beliefs onto this teen rather than consider them to be creating a life on their own terms. Non-monogamy can bring up similar reactions. When people learn that I work with polyamorous folks or when clients in my office begin to explore non-monogamy, I hear some common false beliefs.

Some common judgments I hear include that non-monogamy is unromantic, messy, and selfish. In the therapy room, I encourage people to get curious about where their views of relationships came from. If you were raised on a steady diet of Disney movies and rom-coms, you may have the expectation that finding your "soul mate" will result in your lasting happiness. It can be helpful to understand that the belief "If (X) happens, then I'll be happy" is a seductive trap we can fall into with more than just meeting a romantic partner. This can happen with many socially valued accomplishments, such as getting a promotion at work, buying a new car, or running a marathon. It is important to confront the truth that no person is a happily-ever-after pill, and all rewarding relationships take practice and effort.

> *No person is a happily-ever-after pill, and all rewarding relationships take practice and effort.*

Yes, coordinating more than two schedules can get messy. That being said, with a little extra organization, this can be successfully managed. It has been rumored that Google Calendar was created by a polyamorous person! Planning time together is also a valuable relationship skill that I and many other sex therapists teach their clients that helps contribute to long-term relationship satisfaction.

As for selfishness, I explain to clients that you can be selfish in any relationship style. Heck, you can be selfish as a single person. Effectively navigating non-monogamy means taking ownership of your feelings and prioritizing compassionate communication with your partners. Only you can know what your interpersonal needs are; what is selfish is to assume that it is your partner's responsibility to fulfill all of them.

Although some people think it is impossible to cheat in a non-monogamous relationship, others view non-monogamy as a slippery slope to infidelity and an inevitable breakup. Non-monogamy involves rules or boundaries specific to the relationship, so it is possible to step out of the guidelines set. If you enter into a non-monogamous relationship where you have discussions about your boundaries and expectations, you are already ahead of the game. Often, people enter into monogamous relationships with an unspoken understanding of what those boundaries and expectations are. This can lead to misunderstandings and being more likely to break the rules because you don't know what they are. Good communication about your boundaries in any relationship means you can create a customized relationship that works for you. Security doesn't come from monogamy; security comes from people choosing to be with you because they want to, not because they have to.

> *Security doesn't come from monogamy; security comes from people choosing to be with you because they want to, not because they have to.*

Finally, one of the most common misperceptions of non-monogamy is the belief that jealousy is destructive and impossible to overcome. We will delve further into the physical intensity of the experience of jealousy, its frequent roots in relational trauma, and some coping strategies in chapter 5. For now, I want you to consider whether you have ever experienced jealousy in your own life; whether it was in a monogamous relationship, when dating, or even through friendship or with a coworker. I'm willing to bet that many of you have, because jealousy is a normal human emotion. Non-monogamy may provide more opportunities for jealousy to pop up, simply because you are engaging in more intimate relationships. If someone were experiencing high levels of jealousy while dating monogamously, we wouldn't blame the concept of dating or monogamy; we would look at more specific factors like the quality of the relationships, building emotional distress tolerance, and practicing self-compassion. It is even possible to experience the reverse of jealousy, termed **compersion**, which is a feeling of happiness for your partner's happiness.

Non-Monogamy and Queer Subcultures

A lot of the work on our current understanding of polyamory was built within queer communities before the concept of polyamory gained popularity with straight **cisgender** people in the 1980s and '90s. This makes sense, considering that when a group of people lands outside the dominant cultural narrative for what sex and relationships look like, they are in a position to build it for themselves. As a result, rather than sticking to the heterosexual and monogamous scripts, they can create something new, which can be more malleable to factors like public or group sex, kink, and non-monogamy. It is important for us to dive in, even briefly, to the history of non-monogamy in various queer communities to see how factors such as gender, sexual orientation, and geographic location make for a vast array of experiences.

Casual sex and non-monogamy have been a prominent facet of gay male culture. There is a long history of bathhouses, which became a relatively safe location for men to frequent to have sex with other men, often in groups. These Turkish-style baths became more popular in the first half of the 20th century, and by the 1950s most major cities, including New York and San Francisco, had popular bathhouses that overtly catered to gay men. Over the next two decades, sex and BDSM clubs for gay men were created and grew in popularity as another location for men to meet other men to connect, party, and have sex with.

A RECENT HISTORY
OF POLYAMORY

The earliest form of organized modern non-monogamy grew out of swingers clubs, which were popular with primarily wealthy, white, heterosexual, and bisexual people who lived in the suburbs. These groups started receiving more attention by the media in the 1950s. The groups began secretively, but by the '80s, swingers clubs became easy to find and conventions were bringing in more than 1,000 couples.

The publication of the book *Open Marriage: A New Life Style for Couples* by Nena and George O'Neill in 1984 led to the popularization of the term to mean a marriage that was open to sex with other people, even though the book's primary intention was to emphasize an openness for the couple's growth more broadly than just in the bedroom. The first written proposition of a non-monogamous relationship model that involved more than two egalitarian members (what could now be considered a *line family* or *polycule*) was put forth by Joan and Larry Constantine, who wrote the book *Group Marriage: A Study of Contemporary Multilateral Marriage* in 1974.

Even as North America has decriminalized homosexuality and become a more accepting place for gay men, bathhouses and sex clubs remain popular in the gay male community, speaking to how sex and non-monogamy remain a prominent piece of gay culture.

Prior to the consciousness-raising efforts of the women's movement of the 1960s and '70s, it was difficult for lesbians to meet one another. During this time, cooperatives for lesbian women emerged, and their relationships involved a variety of non-monogamous arrangements. The goal of these living arrangements was for women to find refuge from oppression in order to build lives where they could thrive. They held a community mindset, and everyone contributed to the labor of child care, farming, repairs, and financial planning. The 1980s brought about a divide between differing views within lesbian feminism; however, the valuing of non-monogamy typically remained consistent. Much of the most prominent work discussing polyamory was written by queer women, including authors Hardy and Easton of *The Ethical Slut* and Tristan Taormino of *Opening Up*.

Two queer communities that face discrimination by both heterosexual and homosexual groups are transgender folks and bisexual people. Transgender people face the highest threat of physical violence of the LGBTQ+ identities. This can be as a result of **transphobia**, which refers to negative beliefs, emotions, or actions that discriminate against someone for being trans or not conforming to expected gender roles. **Biphobia** is the term for the same phenomenon but directed at someone who is attracted to more than one gender. Whereas cisgender heterosexual people will never be able to fully understand the lived experiences of trans and bisexual individuals, poly communities are typically very accepting and supportive of these groups. This may contribute to the high prevalence of trans and bi polyamorous people.

New Rights and New Roles

Same-sex marriage has been legal in all 50 states only since 2015. People who fall under the traditionalist wing of the American right have previously argued that marriage equality would be a slippery slope to polygamy, incest, and bestiality. These individuals are typically concerned with upholding the traditional model of the family and worry about any change that might be a threat to it. Fewer people are having children and getting married, which marks a dramatic shift from the nuclear family of the past. Because of this change, living as a queer person brings up obstacles associated with being non-normative, as does living as a non-monogamous person. Non-monogamy and queerness also intersect to create unique challenges.

Legally, it seems, polyamorous people are where gay people were 20 to 30 years ago. In most of the United States, polyamorous relationships have no legal rights: for example, polyamorous people are unable to marry officially, can be denied adoption, can have their children taken away, can be fired, and can be demoted or imprisoned if they are in the military.

Over the past decade, the LGBTQ+ community has grown in its acceptance of ethical non-monogamy, so much so that most cities have queer/poly Meetup and Facebook groups, and polyamorous people are generally included in pride parades. With that said, people who are queer and non-monogamous can face stigma, not only from straight monogamous folks, but also from those who are queer and monogamous. Because LGBTQ+ people have a history of discrimination, there can be implicit and explicit pressures for gay couples to act as role models to legitimize gay marriage. They may worry that bringing non-monogamy into the mix perpetuates the myth that their lifestyle is only about sex, and also that they are to blame for spreading STIs. These pressures are, of course, false, unfair, and further discriminatory. When we look at the high rates of divorce and infidelity in heterosexual marriages, it is clear that they in no way adhere to the same standard. True marriage equality will be achieved only when everyone has permission to suck at marriage equally.

Living in a Monogamous World

In Western culture, monogamy is frequently seen as the default or norm, but what does it really mean to be monogamous? In the discussion around relationship styles, monogamy and non-monogamy can often be presented as opposites. People will often stand rigidly in either the monogamous or non-monogamous camp and argue that one view is morally superior. I encourage you to step back from this black-and-white categorization and indulge the gray.

When we consider what monogamy means, there can be a great variety of definitions. Even the most common understanding of monogamy has changed over time. The definition of monogamy is a socially created concept that at one point implied one sexual relationship for life, and now refers to one sexual relationship at a time (**serial monogamy**). Psychotherapist Esther Perel speaks beautifully about how we are currently at a unique point in history where we expect our partner to provide for us what we once asked for from our entire community. We expect a monogamous partner to be our best friend, co-parent, and fiery lover.

There are a few common struggles I see in sex therapy related to monogamy. First, because society places so much pressure on a monogamous relationship as a sign of status and a signal of happiness, single people can often experience distress and feel like they have failed. It also often means people state that they are monogamous for approval, but are non-consensually non-monogamous in their behavior. I also see couples struggle to find the balance that is needed in a thriving relationship between closeness (which includes safety, trust, and intimacy) and distance (which includes intensity, thrill, and challenge). Many monogamous couples struggle to be sexually compatible. The most common reason couples come to sex therapy is disparity in sexual desire. Couples also often tolerate unsatisfying or painful sex to maintain the status quo or out of fear of losing their partner.

The intention of this book is by no means to pit monogamy against non-monogamy, but rather to encourage the process of self-exploration to see where you can edit out society's expectations to make space for what actually serves you in relationships. In fact, at the time of writing this book, I am in a monogamous relationship. I consider this to be a label that is flexible and can change over time through communication with my partner. This is because relationships evolve, and what works best for me now may not be what I need in the future. Even though monogamy feels like the best fit for me at the moment, the process of breaking down my understanding of relationships to see what messages I internalized from the media, religion, and society, has been some of the most transformational work I have done. I encourage you to do the same. By understanding the influences on your relationship perspectives, you are freed up to decide for yourself what truly works for you and what doesn't.

In your own process of reflecting and untangling these complex themes, I highly recommend therapy, joining poly discussion groups, and reading literature on polyamory, as well as the book *Sex at Dawn* by Christopher Ryan and Cacilda Jethá and anything written by Esther Perel. My favorite explanation of the decision to be monogamous comes from author Christopher Ryan, who compares monogamy to vegetarianism: it is a great option for many reasons, but just because you've made this life decision doesn't mean bacon will stop smelling good.

2

Loving Your Relationship with Sex

We live in a society where the messaging about sex is mixed and confusing. Sex is seen as something dirty, but also as a deeply special act that should be saved for someone you love. Women are bombarded with messages that they need to be the sexual gatekeepers, saying "no" to sex to avoid shame, pain, threats of violence, and diseases. Yet, at the same time, women are expected to be objects of desire by being physically flawless, infinitely orgasmic, and free of inhibitions.

These gendered expectations hurt men as well. Society puts pressure on men to be sexual powerhouses. Men are expected to pursue and conquer. This causes many men to treat sex like a performance and fractures them from experiencing true connection with their partner/s, emotions, and body sensations.

Gender role pressures for men to be dominant and women to be submissive also contribute to miscommunications about consent, as well as high rates of sexual violence. This heteronormative sexual script also leaves trans, genderqueer, and non-binary people completely out of the picture, erasing the value of their sexuality in the public eye. This chapter will encourage you to consider your definition of sex as well as your feelings and fears about it, and attempt to bring to light assumptions you have about sex and where these opinions came from.

What Is Sex?

On the surface, the question "What is sex?" may seem obvious. If you are heterosexual, your initial thought may likely be that it is the act of intercourse, when a penis enters a vagina. In a way you'd be correct, because this is how sex is defined in the dictionary. Is that really all that sex is, though? Isn't that a very narrow definition? Does that mean that if you identify as homosexual, you've never had sex? This definition creates a hierarchy, placing penetrative sex at the top and other behaviors, such as making out, oral sex, and cuddling, as less-than. The consideration that intercourse is the only type of sex is a reflection of the dominant culture that values sex for purposeful reproduction over pleasure.

Many sex therapists, including myself, advocate for broadening what we consider to be sex. I see many of my clients get stuck trying to have the type of sex they think they *should* be having, rather than aiming for the sex that actually feels good for them in the moment. Many people turn sex into something that is goal-oriented and try to achieve a certain number of orgasms, have sex at a particular frequency, or perform what they see in porn. The more outcome-based people become with sex, the more pressure there is, and the less enjoyable the experience is. I work to help my clients shift their intentions with sex: from trying to achieve a particular goal, to allowing themselves to be present with the sensual experience.

> *I work to help my clients shift their intentions with sex: from trying to achieve a particular goal, to allowing themselves to be present with the sensual experience.*

I ask my clients to envision sex as a buffet of options, rather than a pre-ordered meal. Maybe today you feel like some comforting mac-and-cheese, and next time you want some quick and easy chicken wings. When we broaden the definition of what sex is, it becomes about intimacy, play, and connecting. Shifting away from a predetermined sexual script also means building the skills of tuning in to your own body and needs, and communicating them to your partner/s. Many queer and polyamorous people have an easier time ditching the traditional sexual script because they already fall outside the heteronormative box. This means they are more likely to have valuable conversations before sex, communicating their own needs and asking the other person, "Hey, what are you into?" Such a practice can improve everyone's sex life.

Subconscious Assumptions

As a kid, you have very little control over the environment you are brought up in. You have no control over who your parents are, whether they take you to church, what school they send you to, or what news channel they watch over breakfast. Throughout your youth, you are inundated with messages about sex and bodies that you didn't ask for. All this information swirls together to form your assumptions about sex.

Many of your assumptions about sex have been learned from such an early age that they feel like they are a part of you. The good news is that they are not innate, and just as you learned them, you can unlearn them. The first step is to identify which assumptions about sex are no longer serving you, to make space for beliefs that create a happier, healthier, and more fulfilling sex life.

Rarely do people receive **sex-positive** sex education in the United States. There is a wonderful community of sex educators working tirelessly to change this, but at this point, most Americans either receive a curriculum that teaches only abstinence or takes a fear-based approach, focusing solely on avoiding pregnancy and STIs. Yes, it is important to be risk-aware and know how to take measures for safer sex, but an overfocus on the dangers of sex can also lead people to view their bodies and how they decide to use them as degrading and gross. When really, the smells, sounds, and fluids of our bodies are completely normal and beautiful.

When there is inadequate sex education, it is understandable that people turn to porn for their information. Unfortunately, getting sex education from porn is like learning how to drive from watching *The Fast and the Furious*: it can be fun to watch, but definitely does not represent real life. In porn, there is a prescribed set of behaviors that is expected. The heteronormative porn narrative teaches men that sex is their responsibility: They are the sexual initiators and the suppliers of orgasms, they are expected to want sex 24/7 and to get a raging erection on command that lasts for as long as they want. Women are groomed to be objects of desire, to try to mold themselves into an impossibly narrow beauty ideal, and to want the exact right amount of sex. Porn also rarely focuses on female pleasure, and instead typically shows women moaning their way through rough, penetrative sex. In reality, only about 18 percent of women orgasm from penetration alone.

When we limit sexual expression, we repress humanity, perpetuate misinformation, and create a crisis of shame-based sexuality.

It is a tragedy that many people are still told by their communities, families, or churches that there is something wrong with them because of who they love or because of how and when they decide to have sex. There is often a very small set of circumstances in which sex is considered to be okay, which is typically for heterosexual, monogamous, married couples. The social policing of sex hurts everyone. There is as much variability to bodies and sexual behavior as there are people on the planet. When we limit sexual expression, we repress humanity, perpetuate misinformation, and create a crisis of shame-based sexuality. The good news is, even though you didn't have any control of the environment you were brought up in, you do have the power now to decide which beliefs you want to focus on and strengthen, and which to let fall by the wayside.

Your Relationship with Sex

Part of the process of becoming a sex therapist or sex educator is to go through a multiday training called a Sexual Attitude Reassessment

SEX-NEGATIVITY AND
EROTOPHOBIA

Sex-negativity refers to the viewpoint that sexual behavior that is not within the context of marriage or for reproductive purposes is dangerous, deviant, or dirty. There is a long history of sex-negativity within a variety of religious, social, and political groups. In *The Politics of Lust,* John Ince writes about the history of sex-negativity in our culture and how it still shows up today. He also speaks to how sex-negativity contributes to the **erotophobia** in our society, which is the overpowering fear of the harmless sexual expression of ourselves and others.

Erotophobia is prevalent in modern society in a variety of ways. Something is considered to be a phobia if it is not typically dangerous or harmful. This particular phobia is evident in the reactivity to public breastfeeding, nudity (images or in person), talking about sex, use of birth control, sex outside the context of marriage, varieties of sex (e.g., oral, anal, or BDSM), when older people are sexual, porn, and fear of homosexuality (homophobia). Fear and disgust responses to sex are socially learned and perpetuated. Take, for example, the aversion to the perfectly healthy, natural, and pleasurable behavior of masturbation. If someone grows up being told this behavior is shameful, they will begin to believe it. Sometimes kids get caught by their parents while touching their genitals without realizing what they are doing, and if the parent responds in a way that is judgmental, angry, or punitive, this will trigger a fear response from the limbic system and the brain will code this behavior as "dangerous," perpetuating an aversive response in the future.

(or SAR). During the SAR, people are exposed to challenging topics in the realm of sexuality and are provided with a supportive environment to process their emotional reactions. The purpose of this intense experience is to unearth, confront, and examine existing assumptions and negative associations about sexual topics in order to better understand and limit our own judgments so we can provide our clients with the best help we can.

People who attend an SAR are generally sex-positive, and even so, almost everyone has an intense emotional reaction to pieces of the material, and many break down and cry at some point (I was a mess!). Sex is a charged topic, and we are often unaware of the areas where we hold automatic negative associations. When you make a conscious effort to examine your automatic negative judgments, you might find that your reaction shifts. Whereas attending a SAR is a powerful experience, there are other ways to examine your relationship to sex through reading, journaling, joining a discussion group, and, of course, therapy.

In sex therapy, a lot of the early work is to help the client understand the factors that have influenced their current relationship with sex. People will speak to their past relationships, religion, cultural influences, medical histories, mental health factors, and body image struggles.

I ask people to think back to how they felt when they decided to have consensual sex for the first time. Sometimes people felt excited and in love, and others felt worried it would hurt or were afraid of being judged. This can provide insight into the early messaging that was internalized about sex. I will always ask clients about their family of origin, including how affection was shown, what intimacy looked and felt like, how pleasure was approached, and what messages they received about sex. Our early experiences in our families affect us both positively and negatively in obvious and subtle ways, particularly with sex.

Seek to connect with sexuality in a way that feels safe to you: read a book, listen to a podcast, take a class, venture into a sex shop! Sexuality is a healthy and integral part of life.

Exploring Messages about Sex

Divide a piece of paper into four quadrants. Label the four boxes "friends," "family," "community," and "society." Spend time with each quadrant free writing all the messages that come to mind that you received from each group about sex. For both the "friends" and the "family" categories, reflect on what was modeled as well as what was explicitly said. For "community," consider factors like the neighborhood you grew up in, any extracurricular activities you were a part of, and whether you attended a place of worship. For the broader "society" category, think about the influences, pressures, and expectations put upon you based on your gender, race, sexual orientation, appearance, neurodiversity, socioeconomic status, physical capabilities, and geographic location. You may then wish to go through your list with a pen and a highlighter, highlight messages you would like to keep, and cross out the messages you would like to let go of.

I often hear from clients that their parents never talked to them about sex. This frustrates some, and others brush it off and say something like, "But if I'd asked, they would have told me."

But how is it fair to put children in charge of their own learning about sex? When parents don't talk about sex, three big messages people can get include: sex is shameful, their body is something to be afraid of, or sex is too indulgent and not worth spending time on. If this matches your experience, the good news is that you can start to re-parent yourself as an adult. Start by noticing what beliefs you learned growing up and one you now hold about sex. Honor the wounding caused by a household radio silence on sexuality. It does not mean your parents are bad people or that they intended to cause harm. Seek to connect with sexuality in a way that feels safe to you: read a book, listen to a podcast, take a class, venture into a sex shop. Sexuality is a healthy and integral part of life.

Sex-Positivity

Sex-positivity is an accepting and nonjudgmental viewpoint about sex, in which all consensual sexual behavior with oneself and others is seen as a healthy part of the human experience. Personal freedom is highly valued, whether it is of sexual expression, feelings, or fantasies. The sex-positivity movement supports a variety of topics related to human sexuality, including reproductive rights, safer sex, gender identity, sexual orientation, sex education, polyamory, body acceptance, BDSM/kink, and asexuality. The World Health Organization defines sexual health as a "state of mental and social well-being in relation to sexuality; it is not merely the absence of disease, dysfunction, or infirmity."

Although the term existed previously, the sex-positivity movement was first prominent during the sociopolitical sexual liberation movement of the 1960s and '70s. This time saw certain groups displaying a more positive attitude toward the use of contraception, public nudity, legalizing abortion, interracial marriage, gay rights, and feminism. It was said that this was a time of normalizing masturbation, sexual fantasies, premarital sex, and porn.

From the sexual liberation movement through today, a lot of the work promoting sex-positivity has been done by women—particularly queer women and/or women of color, such as Stormé DeLarverie, Marsha P. Johnson, and Audre Lorde. A large piece of the sex positivity movement is reclaiming sexuality and pleasure as an essential piece of mental and physical well-being for all people, regardless of factors such as race, gender, or sexual orientation. This is revolutionary work because in the Western world, the sexual template we are shown consists of thin, white, cisgender, heterosexual couples who have sex for

AFFIRMATIONS FOR
SEX-POSITIVE THINKING

We often have to make a concerted effort to fight the sex-negative messaging we received as a result of growing up in our culture. Internalized sex-negativity may show up in surprising ways, whether through disgust toward certain body parts or bodily functions, cutting yourself off from feeling sexual desire, or judgment around expression of your own sexuality. When you start shifting toward a more sex-positive attitude, it is inevitable that you will experience some competing thoughts (or cognitive dissonance). This can feel uncomfortable, but it's actually a good thing because when you're aware of your competing views, you can start to choose which view you'd like to foster and which you'd like to let fall by the wayside. Positive affirmations can be a helpful way to strengthen and grow your own sex-positivity.

→ I am deserving of pleasure.
→ Pleasure is healing.
→ Pleasure is freedom.
→ I am free to indulge my desires.
→ It is a powerful thing to own my desires.

reproductive purposes; anyone who does not fit into this category is ignored, suppressed, or hyper- or hypo-sexualized.

There is often a lot of overlap between the people doing work in the sex-positivity movement and the fat acceptance movement. Sonya Renee Taylor, the writer of *The Body Is Not an Apology*, is a prominent voice advocating for radical self-love, which means believing in your inherent value as a human being and ditching society's hierarchy that places thin, white, able bodies above all else. adrienne maree brown is also a powerful voice in the world of sex-positivity and body acceptance. Her book *Pleasure Activism* is a wonderful resource speaking to the essential role that pleasure plays in our lives and the importance of historically disenfranchised groups reclaiming pleasure (whether through food, rest, or sex) as a daily practice.

Consent

Content Warning: The next section will address the topic of sexual violence. Although I believe this is an invaluable topic, it is a heavy one. If you notice yourself becoming too activated (e.g., thoughts racing, heart pounding, mentally checking out), this reaction may be a sign that this is a section to skip for now. That is perfectly fine. In fact, it is a sign of strength to be able to show that level of awareness and self-compassion. We do our best learning when we are on the edge of discomfort; if we are fully overwhelmed and flooded, we are no longer benefiting ourselves. If this section brings up challenging feelings, do what you need to do to be kind to yourself: consider going for a walk around the block, grabbing a cup of tea, or listening to your favorite playlist. This chapter will be here when you're ready.

The national conversation on consent has shifted since October 2017 with the beginning of the #MeToo movement. The movement caught fire when Tarana Burke's phrase was tweeted by an actress and people used the hashtag to proclaim over social media that they had been sexually harassed or assaulted. Since then, more than 1.7 million people in 85 countries have tweeted "#MeToo." The #MeToo movement was considered to be so influential that *Time* magazine named the "Silence Breakers," referring to the people who spoke out about their sexual assault experiences, their 2017 Person of the Year. The #MeToo movement significantly increased media attention and opened up a nationwide discussion on sexual assault and consent.

> *An essential skill of being an ethical slut is to know your own sexual boundaries and respond respectfully to the boundaries of others.*

An essential skill of being an ethical slut is to know your own sexual boundaries and respond respectfully to the boundaries of others. This next section will highlight how practicing consent will empower you to respectfully address your needs and those of your partner/s. Consent is a clear, enthusiastic, "Yes!," which can be taken back at any time, and is given without the presence of coercion, force, or intoxication. To engage in ethical sex and relationships, consent is essential.

Unwanted Sexual Activity

It is an unfortunate reality that a discussion about sex also warrants a discussion about sexual trauma. Sexual assault is defined as any unwanted sexual activity, including both unwelcome touching (e.g., kissing, fondling, or grabbing) and violent acts. A very low rate of people report their sexual assaults, so a conservative estimate is that one in five women and one in 71 men will be raped in their lifetime.

Although anyone can be sexually assaulted, it is important to know that people in more marginalized groups, such as disabled people, sex workers, LGBTQ+ folks, and people of color, experience much higher rates of sexual violence. This goes to show that in sex, there are power dynamics at play. To practice ethical sexual relationships, bring awareness to your own positionality and that of your partner/s. Know that if you are in a more powerful position, your partner may not feel as comfortable speaking up if they feel uneasy during sex. Know that you can handle more of the responsibility to check in with your partner for ongoing consent, and that this will help create more safety and security in the relationship.

Verbal vs. Nonverbal

There's no denying that it can be difficult to communicate feelings of discomfort during a sexual interaction. Consent needs to be specific and enthusiastic. People can communicate this verbally and nonverbally. Many factors make communicating clear consent more challenging, including social pressures (particularly for women) to be compliant, to be polite, and not to hurt anyone's feelings. Past sexual and relational trauma can also influence how people respond in a sexual scenario.

When people have past traumatic sexual experiences, sex can be coded in our brains as a "threat." People respond to these threats in different ways according to the stress response that our bodies believe to be best in each particular scenario. We will talk more about our bodies' stress responses through the lens of polyvagal theory in chapter 7.

Most people are familiar with the concept of going into "fight-or-flight" mode, but it is also important to note that our stress responses can include a "freeze" response. If someone is freezing, this may look like zoning out, speaking very little, or having difficulty responding to questions. There is also a learned behavior that can emerge called a "fawn" or "tend and befriend" response. A placate reaction typically looks like acting extra agreeable and going with the flow of what is happening so as not to ruffle any feathers. Both the freeze and fawn are common responses for sexual assault survivors to slip into, and it can be helpful to learn your own signs of slipping into a trauma response as well as those of your sexual partner.

Unconsciousness and Intoxication

I wish I didn't have to write this next sentence, but I do. It is not possible to consent to sex if you or your partner is unconscious or drunk. This explanation is necessary because it is not uncommon for people to be intoxicated or unconscious when they are sexually assaulted. When I give presentations to colleges about understanding, preventing, and responding to sexual assault, I show a scene from the 1984 John Hughes romantic comedy *Sixteen Candles*. The clip depicts two teenage boys, one the established heartthrob and the other a nerd. The heartthrob is offering his car to the nerd to take his girlfriend home to have sex with her, because she is passed out from drinking. Cut to the next scene, where the nerd carries the girlfriend to the car, her body slung over his shoulder like a slain deer.

This scene typically elicited a strong response from the groups I presented to. The faculty who were old enough to remember the film when it came out would express shock; they recalled previously laughing at the film, not thinking twice about the severe boundary violations shown in that scene. In the several decades since this film came out, and partially thanks to the #MeToo movement, we now have a deeper understanding that this is not an example of consensual sexual behavior.

Affirmative Consent and "Yes Means Yes"

You always need an enthusiastic "yes!" for any form of sexual touching, whether it is intercourse, making out, or a slap on the ass. The absence of a "no" does not suffice, and if someone demonstrates body language or body posture that suggests they are afraid or uninterested, that would not be considered **enthusiastic consent**. Consent is ongoing, which means it is necessary for sexual partners to check in with each other, because it is also perfectly fine for it to be taken back at any time. This also means that if people have had sex previously, it does not mean that they are an automatic "yes" for the future.

Consent is ongoing, which means it is necessary for sexual partners to check in with each other, because it is also perfectly fine for it to be taken back at any time.

It is important that everyone engaging in the sexual activity is aware of what specifically they are consenting to. For example, saying yes to a kiss does not mean that oral sex is also agreed upon. For consent to be present, everyone also needs to be honest. For instance, if one person has said they will use a condom, and they do not (or they remove it) without telling their sexual partner, that is not consent.

Overcoming Sexual Trauma

Sexual trauma is a common and devastating event. If you've been impacted by sexual trauma and are feeling ready to process some of this hurt, talking with a therapist can be a powerful and transformative experience. Sharing your story in a way that feels safe to you, whether through speaking with a therapist, journaling, or talking with a trusted friend, can be an empowering way to reclaim your own experience. Shame breeds in silence, but cannot survive when your story is witnessed, validated, and supported. I have yet to meet a survivor who did not at one point blame themselves for the experience. It is heart-breaking, yet understandable when you consider how our society at large too often criticizes, blames, and disbelieves survivors.

Shame breeds in silence, but cannot survive when your story is witnessed, validated, and supported.

To the survivors: Know that the guilt and self-doubt are insidious and brutal. Know that what you are feeling is a natural reaction to a terrible thing you experienced that nobody should ever have to go through. **It was not your fault.** You did not ask for what happened to you. Find people who can remind you of this. You will need to hear this over and over again. I know how this can break you open and change your whole life. I also want you to know that you show incredible strength. If you take the time to feel your pain and take care of yourself, you will come out of this backbreaking work not necessarily "healed," but inevitably more resilient and self-understanding than you could ever imagine.

Pathologizing

The tendency for our culture to normalize male sexual aggression and sexual violence, and particularly against women and marginalized groups, is referred to as **rape culture**. It is a continuum of threatened violence that ranges from sexual remarks to sexual touching to rape itself. When there is an acceptance or lack of action against sexual violence, the importance of consent is neglected, or the severe impact of rape is joked about, rape culture continues.

There are some common misconceptions about the occurrence of sexual assault, which also perpetuate judgment and victim-blaming attitudes toward survivors. For example, we tell women to avoid being alone at night in parking lots or alleys, when factually most sexual assaults occur in a private home. It is also true that 82 percent of sexual assaults are perpetrated by someone the survivor knows.

To combat the rape culture we live in, it is important to believe survivors and avoid blaming them. You have been influenced, as we all have, by the many myths surrounding sexual assault. It is never the survivor's fault. Know that the survivor is the expert on their own experience. If you are assisting someone who has been assaulted, the best thing you can do is provide acceptance and support as they find their own path to healing and justice.

Resources

The path to healing from sexual trauma involves establishing a feeling of safety in the body, as well as the mind. One of the most helpful books for understanding the impact of trauma as well as how to move past it is *The Body Keeps the Score* by Bessel van der Kolk. As the title of the book suggests, much of the impact of trauma is felt in the body; this can mean that even years later, when a survivor is in a safe situation, their nervous system can still be on high alert. For this reason, it can be beneficial to go through therapies that engage the body as well as the mind.

Some body-based therapies that are helpful for sexual assault survivors include eye movement desensitization and reprocessing (EMDR), somatic experiencing, art therapy, and trauma-sensitive yoga. "Trauma-informed" has become a bit of a buzzword in the therapy world, so when selecting a practitioner it can be helpful to ask the therapist what their particular experience is in working with sexual trauma and what approach they use. The Rape, Abuse & Incest National Network (RAINN) is an organization that has various resources for coping with a sexual assault experience. Survivors can also get immediate one-time virtual crisis sessions with the nonprofit organization Resilience.

Some other helpful books include:

You Can't Own the Fucking Stars by Clementine Morrigan

I Hope We Choose Love: A Trans Girl's Notes from the End of the World by Kai Cheng Thom

The Gifts of Imperfection by Brené Brown

Self-Compassion by Kristin Neff

3

Honoring Your
Needs and Fears

You need to love yourself before you love can love anyone else. I'm calling bullshit. Although I do agree that learning to turn toward yourself with care and compassion is an invaluable practice, this popular statement makes it sound like *loving yourself* is a destination you arrive at, when really it is a lifelong process—and yes, the deeper we learn to love ourselves, the deeper we can love others.

Paradoxically, we *also* can learn to love ourselves by being in relationships with others. We are social beings; our brains are literally wired for connection. The limbic system in our brain is also referred to as our *mammalian brain*. It is aptly named because the need we have for touch and intimacy is also present in other mammals. To see this in action, type in my personal favorite Internet search, "animals being friends," for an adorable array of cuddly pals. What sets humans apart, however, is that we have the ability to become aware of our own sex and relationship needs and insecurities and the ability to communicate them to others.

When I bring up the topic of relationship needs and fears with my clients, people usually have one of two reactions. They either feel that they are "too needy" or believe they don't have any relationship needs; ironically, these people are often in relationships with each other. Two truths here are: (1) human needs are universal and (2) you are only as "needy" as your unmet needs. This next section will help you explore and identify some core needs for you in your relationship/s.

45

Taking Responsibility for Your Needs

Whatever perspective you're coming from when you opened this book, getting clear on your relationship needs is incredibly valuable. It can be particularly helpful to consider the question, "Why am I interested in ENM?" As well as, "What makes the challenges of ENM worth it for me?" When you think back on the previous chapters, reflect on what components of ENM get you excited. There is so much variation in ENM, it is important to reflect on what exactly you are looking for. Are you looking for the novelty of sex? Are you attempting to maintain the structure of your existing relationship as much as possible, but just soften the restrictions a bit? Or perhaps you are looking to adopt a relationship anarchy perspective.

In any case, a great place to start is to identify your relationship values and needs. A common phrase in the couples therapy world is "You are responsible for your own needs." This is a bit misleading because it's sort of true, but not quite. What is true is that only you know what your needs are, and only you can be the one to ask for them to be met in your relationship. This is a skill that requires practice, building emotional intelligence and self-understanding. What's not true is that you have to fulfill all your needs yourself. In fact, it's not possible, because we are social beings. With that said, once you identify and communicate your needs, though they are more likely to be met this way, you also cannot expect that your partner/s will fulfill *all* of them.

> *Only you know what your needs are, and only you can be the one to ask for them to be met in your relationship.*

Whether you have one, two, or six partners, sometimes your needs won't get met, and that is okay. As you develop awareness of your needs, it is also helpful to build a variety of strategies to meet them. Healthy relationships are not selfish *or* selfless when it comes to needs, but rather there is an equal valuing of the needs of your partner/s as well as your own. This interdependence is not a sign of weakness, but rather a sign of strength through vulnerability and heightened connection.

Balancing Sexual Needs

Getting our sexual needs met in relationships is often challenging because we frequently find ourselves in the middle of competing desires. For sexual relationships, we want both excitement and stability. By excitement I mean that we want thrill, heat, and intensity. This feeling is built through a longing for one another, and longing can only happen when there is a separateness. This feeling is often present at the beginning of a relationship. It is frequently called romantic love, and it's what we think of when we imagine dizzying teenage infatuation. In poly circles, this is also often termed **new relationship energy (NRE)**, referring to the phase where you obsessively think about the other person and you can't keep your hands off each other. Often people look back on that time of their lives quite fondly. But there's also a downside to this intensity, because the fieriness is a result of a lack of stability, security, and trust. It can be interesting to consider how we don't actually need safety or trust in order to have hot sex in relationships. A dark example of this is that studies of women who have been in abusive relationships have shown that some of their best sexual experiences happened after violent acts.

The other side to this paradox of desire is that we also want deep connection and intimacy in our sexual relationships. These qualities often show up in longer-term relationships because it takes time for trust to build. Sometimes the result of this is the extinguishing of sexual desire. In my work, I see this in partners who come in saying, "We're best friends, but we feel more like roommates than a couple." This is an example of people who have a really strong bond, but struggle to weave in eroticism, seduction, and playfulness. Esther Perel's book *Mating in Captivity* is devoted to unraveling this tension between the need for attachment and differentiation. She writes about how there is space for both exciting fantasy and intimate connection, just maybe not at the same time. She writes about how the couples who are able

How Do You Identify Your Sexual Needs?

A great place to start can be to go through a *yes-no-maybe* list of questions about sexual things you'd like to try. I recommend taking time to reflect on what fantasies you often have. It can be helpful to number a page from 1 to 20 and then, without thinking too hard, write out 20 fantasies. Our fantasies are far from frivolous. In fact, our fantasies serve as a way to work through our deepest desires. Beneath our fantasies and typically beneath our level of awareness, what we long for can serve as a gateway to understanding our unmet needs.

For example, imagine a woman who is a hard-working accountant. When she gets home for the day, she reads *Game of Thrones* fan fiction and fantasizes about elaborate character role-play with her girlfriend. She keeps this fantasy close to her chest out of embarrassment when, really, she doesn't have anything to be embarrassed about. Our fantasies do not necessarily represent what we want in real life, but are instead a gateway to understanding themes around our sexual desires and unmet needs. In this example, the accountant's unmet need may be that of creativity or playfulness. This makes sense, given that she spends a lot of her time trying to meet expectations and follow protocols. The wonderful thing about sexual relationships is that it provides an opportunity to meet needs for one another that go deeper than physical release.

DON SHARES A FANTASY

Don (pronouns: he/him) arrived at his first therapy session madly in love, but worried. He was six months into a new relationship and talked about how he had found his *person*. What he was concerned about, however, was that he was feeling an increasing need to address an unmet sexual need of his. He desired to put on a dress and makeup before having sex with his girlfriend, Jess. He spoke to how freeing and exciting it was for him to express himself in this way, but how he had never felt safe enough to do so with anyone else. He now felt hopeful that Jess would be open to it, because so far she had proven to be curious, kind, and open-minded about sex.

In helping Don to prepare for this conversation, I let him know that it was understandable for him to feel nervous talking to Jess, and that it would also be okay if the conversation felt uncomfortable. We aren't typically taught how to have these conversations about sex, so it is a brave thing to be vulnerable and share a fantasy with someone. I normalized how in our sexual relationships we will never 100 percent match up with our partners in terms of what turns us on. So, it would be fine if Don's dressing up were not as exciting for Jess as it was for him. As long as the activity didn't make her feel completely uncomfortable or unsafe, a great sexual partner is someone who is keen to hear your sexual desires, will listen without judgment, and is down to help you get off. Fortunately for Don, Jess fit the bill of a great sexual partner, and although it didn't necessarily arouse her, it did bring her satisfaction to support something that brought Don so much pleasure.

to balance these forces understand that it is normal for desire to go in phases, and it's okay to have times where sex is less prominent, but that if the couple still values pleasure and an erotic life that is broader than sex, the passion will resurface.

The methods people choose to navigate this paradox will differ. Some non-monogamous people will choose to have different types of relationships to fill these needs. For example, someone may have a more trusting relationship with someone they are married to or raise kids with, and have pleasant, connected sex with this person; and then they may seek excitement and novelty through a variety of other relationships. Someone who desires to remain monogamous may bring more thrill into their relationship by having sex in different locations, with new toys or role-play.

Communicating Your Needs

Say it louder for the people in the back: everyone has needs in relationships! There are many needs that are considered universal, such as physical well-being, freedom, acceptance, closeness, self-expansion, and self-esteem. Many factors influence what needs show up for us in particular relationships. Often, whether something was scarce for us in our childhood influences how much we value this need now. For example, if someone grew up with an overbearing mother, they might highly value autonomy in their adult relationships.

Where it can get tricky is that we tend to assume that what is important to us is also of the same degree of importance to our partner/s. If you've ever read Gary Chapman's *The Five Love Languages*, it's a similar idea. For example, if you feel most loved when you receive gifts, you will most often show love by giving gifts, when your partner might actually feel the most loved by getting a nice big smooch.

My favorite simple workaround for expressing your needs is this: Rate your need from 1 to 10. When you make a request from a partner, start to normalize the conversation around asking how important it is to them. You will quickly see how different your needs can be. For example, with my partner, it's important to me that he is by my side at big life events. So, having him show up to my thesis defense was a 10/10 for me.

I remember being quite shocked when I learned a 7 or 8 for him was to keep the kitchen organized (typically a low priority for me). The second part of this is to understand that expressing a need is always a request and never a demand. If you or your partner rates anything a 6/10 or higher, and the other person declines, it just means that a conversation should be had about why they are making this decision. When you begin to normalize the needs conversation in your relationship/s, you can make huge strides to better understand and support each other.

People over Needs

Within monogamous relationships, it is not uncommon for people to expect one person to fulfill all their needs, whether it be for passion, deep conversation, or salsa dancing. Some people have become aware of the impossibility of one person being everything for them and turn to polyamory as the solution. People still run into trouble here, because humans are not need-filling machines. Some needs are straightforward, like the salsa partner, but most people are talking about much more nuanced and abstract qualities, such as a need for personal growth or excitement.

If people do attempt to add partners in response to filling needs, there is the risk of filling your relationship capacity before you fill your needs. It is common for people to overestimate how much their needs will be met and drastically underestimate how much they will be required to give in their relationships. Let's say you have seven intense needs in your life: Could you imagine maintaining seven deep relationships? That would be challenging for most people to manage. At a certain point, more partners can also be a strategy to avoid intimacy rather than cultivate it.

Societal factors (e.g., race, class, access to health care) and individual factors (e.g., mental illness, neurodiversity, trauma history) impact what we need and what we have to offer. For example, consider a polycule in which one partner is in a wheelchair, another has ADHD, and the third person has complex posttraumatic stress disorder. Would it be fair to expect an equal exchange of what is given and what is received among the three partners? Of course not. Equity, rather than equality, should be the goal. **Equality** is based on a false understanding that everyone has the same needs. **Equity**, on the other hand, is the expectation that every partner should have the right to ask for what they need and to have the opportunity for that need to be met.

Feeling Insecure

Moments of insecurity can flare up regardless of what relationship structure you are in. I often hear from folks in monogamous relationships that they would feel too anxious in an ethically non-monogamous relationship. From polyamorous people, I hear that sometimes when they feel insecure, they can unfairly judge themselves for being "bad at being poly." We often want to avoid and resist uncomfortable emotions. It can be a helpful reminder for all of us that feelings are not good or bad. All emotions—even the sticky ones like worry, fear, anger, and jealousy—carry information. You have not failed if you feel insecure or unsafe in a relationship.

> *All emotions—even the sticky ones like worry, fear, anger, and jealousy—carry information. You have not failed if you feel insecure or unsafe in a relationship.*

Many different factors influence our sense of security in relationships. In chapter 7, we will explore **attachment theory**, which speaks to how our early caregivers influence how we interact in relationships as adults. For now, it is important to take a moment to acknowledge how societal factors influence our feeling of stability in relationships, because there is a tendency to pathologize the individual. This is particularly clear with mental health challenges; for example, in how we diagnose anorexia rather than considering media pressures, sexism, or diet culture; in how we label someone with borderline personality disorder rather than looking at their attachment trauma; and in how we ask "Why do transgender people have such high rates of depression?" rather than exploring widespread transphobia.

We are social beings influenced by the environment. Our culture sets us up to have a dysfunctional sense of self-worth. We are sold the belief that our relationship security depends on whether we make six figures, rock a hot bod, and are orgasm machines. Because of this pressure, it is understandable that we learn to base our worth on external factors. This tendency leads to a fragile sense of self-worth, competitiveness, comparison, and a feeling that love is scarce.

Confronting Your Insecurities

It is important to consider how feelings of insecurity are not an individual failing. With that said, it is also helpful to look at some strategies for how to cope with the acute moments of discomfort.

Reminders of Your Emotional Resilience

In moments when insecurity rears its ugly head, it can be helpful to have a touchstone of phrases to remind you of your own emotional resilience.

→ It's okay to not be okay.
→ I'm allowed to ask for what I need.
→ My emotions are valid.
→ I can feel hard feelings.
→ I have the tools I need to cope.
→ I am loved and valued beyond my romantic relationship/s.
→ Regardless of whether this relationship works out, I will be okay.
→ I am deserving of a partner and community that make space for my needs.
→ Right now, as I am, I am worthy of love.

Insecurities can show up as thoughts (e.g., defensiveness, mind racing, self-criticism), emotions (fear, jealousy, anger), or body sensations (tightness in chest, difficulty sleeping or eating, heart racing). Harsh thoughts release stress hormones and put your body into fight-or-flight mode. It is challenging to think clearly when you are in this state, so it is important to help move your body through the stress response. This can be done through exercise, connecting with your support system, or caring for yourself in a way that feels nurturing (such as a hot shower, putting on your favorite lotion, or cooking yourself a nice meal). All these activities send signals to your brain that it can stop sounding the alarm bells because you are safe.

Building Security

It is valuable to address insecurity by turning toward it with calm curiosity. Explore what it's trying to protect you from by being on high alert for danger or highlighting your perceived flaws. Ask this insecure part of yourself what it needs. Sometimes this part is recognizing a present threat. If you are feeling frequently insecure in your relationship, this may be a sign that a boundary is being crossed, that there's an unmet need to express, or possibly, that this relationship isn't a good fit for you. At other times, the hypervigilance may be a result of past relationship hurt from your parents or former romantic partners. You may want to ask yourself, "Is this a relationship problem or something going on inside me?" Regardless of whether it is a response to a past or present threat, the emotional experience is equally valid. What differs is whether it is something for you to process and address within yourself, or if it is something to address through making changes in the relationship.

In addition to checking in with the insecurity and asking what it needs, you may also want to try sending love to the part of you that is feeling insecure. If you can imagine it, turn toward the insecurity as though it were a separate character within you (maybe a younger version of yourself), and thank it for keeping you safe from whatever it believes you need to be protected from. The big secret of insecurity is that it is usually rooted in fear, so much so that this part of you forgets all the times you overcame hard things in the past. So, let this part of you know that you have support and strategies to handle emotional pain. Regardless of whether this relationship works out, you will be okay, even if it hurts for a while. You are resilient.

> *The big secret of insecurity is that it is usually rooted in fear, so much so that this part of you forgets all the times you overcame hard things in the past.*

Confronting Fears

People tend to approach fears in relationships in one of two ways. Some experience the threat of fear as an alarm bell and respond through attempts to predict, control, and solve. Others detach from the fear through denying, numbing, or pushing it away. Both are attempts to deal with the same unavoidable risks that come with the territory of loving as human beings. When we resort to either of these threat management tendencies, it is not possible to connect with our partners or be present with what is actually happening in the moment. All relationship structures face these risks; however, people in ethically non-monogamous relationships may be faced with them more frequently or at a higher intensity, simply because there are more people in the mix.

Although we all will dip into unproductive strategies from time to time, particularly when our relationship security is threatened, we also have the ability to learn how to hold steady through the fear. We all have tendencies that characterize how we respond when our relationship security is threatened; these are called "attachment styles," which we will dig into further in chapter 7. Briefly, when we are feeling insecure in our relationships, we often respond with behaviors that are considered to be more "anxious" (i.e., intimacy seeking) or more "avoidant" (i.e., distancing). For people who tend to be more anxious in relationships (e.g., struggle to directly communicate needs, "act out" to make a partner jealous, bombard with texts), it is valuable to learn how to soothe

BILLIE CONFRONTS
RELATIONSHIP INSECURITIES

Billie (pronouns: they/them) struggled with feelings of insecurity when their partner went on dates. This was a new feeling for them, because in their past polyamorous relationships they felt fully comfortable and even excited when their primary partner made new romantic connections. Now, when Billie's partner is on a date, they feel so physically stressed they are unable to fall asleep or eat. They began to reflect on what factors were causing their body to have such a strong physical response.

They put the pieces together and realized that at the same time they began dating their current partner, their parents were going through a divorce. Billie realized that their parents' divorce was bringing up past abandonment pain they had felt as a child. They were relieved to make this connection because they realized that although their partner's dates were a trigger for their stress response, it was not the cause.

Now, when Billie notices themself feeling emotionally flooded, they think of their young self and they speak to them with compassion. They validate themself by saying things like, "It was so hard when you felt abandoned in that moment" and "It's okay to have these feelings." They have practice identifying their needs in these tough moments, as well as making requests of their partner when there is something they can do to help. They have found it helpful to have a place to process feelings with their partner before dates. Another strategy has been to cultivate intimacy in their friendships, to remind themself that they are loved and safe beyond their romantic relationship. They schedule platonic sleepovers with friends on evenings when their partner has dates so they have a place to share whatever feelings come up for them during that time period.

your nervous system when it is flooded and to bolster a sense of security and safety, both in yourself and outside your romantic relationship. If you generally use more avoidant strategies (e.g., overly self-reliant, downplays the importance of relationships, "ghosting"), it is important to notice when you are pulling away as a protective mechanism, and in those moments practice vulnerability through identifying and expressing your emotions to your partner/s. Rewiring these patterns in moments of stress is not easy, but just like a truck driving through a field, the more frequently the truck drives over a new path, the easier it will become over time to follow it.

Loss

Sorry to get dark here, but one thing we can count on is that all relationships end, whether through breakups or death. Everyone would agree that the loss of a loved one is unimaginably painful. Heartbreak, on the other hand, I consider to be the most agonizing human experience that is most frequently trivialized. It is ironic, because anyone who has ever gone through a major breakup can attest to the fact that it feels *physically* painful. I have had clients go to the doctor because they couldn't imagine how an emotional experience could cause such a searing hurt. I honestly believe we should have paid leave for heartbreak.

> *Loss is part of loving, and you can withstand the pain of it. You can handle the hard feelings.*

There is actually an explanation for why it hurts so damn much. Our early experiences with our parents and caregivers affect how we relate romantically later in life. Our maps for intimate relationships (or **attachment styles**) are formed at a time when the end of a relationship would actually be a life-or-death experience. If, for example, your parents decided to up and leave when you were five years old, you would have serious concerns for your survival. This threat becomes hardwired into your brain so that as an adult, you experience the same visceral emotional response to abandonment even though you now have the strategies to continue living. So, it is understandable that we try to do everything we can to avoid this type of loss. Yet, when faced with the fear of a relationship ending, it is important to remind yourself that this should not be a barrier to loving. Loss is part of loving, and you can withstand the pain of it. You can handle the hard feelings.

Being Alone

My first relationship began when I was in high school and went on for seven years. When that relationship ended, I was single for the first time in my adult life, and I was terrified of feeling lonely. I was also forced to confront how much I had pointed to my relationship status for an external measure of success and a sense of security.

> *There is no one right path to meaningful connection in our lives. It is okay to feel lonely.*

I am not alone in this fear of *being* alone. We attempt to avoid loneliness because it is uncomfortable, and because being in a relationship is perceived as a measure of success in our society, being single can be seen as a failure. In my early 20s, I had fully bought into these expectations. However, in the process of being alone, I was able to reread the memo I had gotten from society about how my life should look. I had the epiphany that how closely our Facebook timelines match up with our friends' is no indication of how fulfilled we are in our lives. There is no one right path to meaningful connection in our lives. It is okay to feel lonely. Loneliness is a human emotion that can show up if you are single, if you are married, and even if you have multiple relationships. As always, emotions are information, so it can be rewarding to check in with the loneliness and ask what it is trying to tell you.

Being Uncomfortable

It is actually healthy to experience discomfort in our relationships from time to time. For any of us who have ever taken an exercise class, we have heard that *change happens at the edge of our comfort zone.* Regardless of how annoying this can be to hear when you're thinking you might actually be holding a plank for the rest of eternity, this is one of those cheesy sayings that's repeated again and again because it's true. Being at the *edge* of discomfort is an important distinction here, because you never want to be so overwhelmed that you shut down (or hurt your back while planking).

We grow when we are able to sit with uncomfortable experiences with nonjudgmental curiosity. One of the most valuable pieces of being in a relationship is that the other person is there to hold up a mirror to you about your own behavior so you can learn your blind spots. Through your relationships, you can become more intimately acquainted with your fears, insecurities, and triggers. When we gain further insight into these challenging experiences, the grip they hold over us can loosen, and we gain awareness into how we may want to change our responses to them in the future.

Is Ethical Non-Monogamy Right for Me?

Only you are able to determine what your relationship needs are, and only you can communicate them to others. Because our partners will not always be able to meet our needs, it is beneficial to find multiple ways of meeting them. For example, if you have a need for deep conversation, sometimes your partner will be too tired to provide that for you. On these days, you may turn to someone else to speak with, or to other activities like journaling or therapy.

Our sexual needs in relationships can often be boiled down to a need for either excitement or security. These needs often compete with each other, and there are an infinite number of ways to navigate this paradox. Some decide to infuse novelty within a monogamous relationship, and others may approach this through variations of ENM. In sexual relationships, it is also completely normal to differ from your partner/s regarding some of your interests. To maximize sexual satisfaction in relationships, it is helpful to be willing to fulfill the other person's fantasies that you have slightly positive or neutral feelings

Am I Ready? Reflection

1. Why choose ENM?

2. What arrangement of ENM feels like the best fit for me?

3. What are my top relationship values, and how does ENM align with them?

4. What makes me feel fulfilled in a sexual relationship?

5. How do I want to feel in my relationship/s?

6. What scares me the most about ENM?

7. What challenges do I anticipate with ENM?

8. What role do I want to have in my partners' lives?

9. How do I envision my partner's role in my life? If I have more than one partner, would their roles be different?

10. What meaning would ENM give to my life?

toward. This is just like how it is beneficial from time to time to let your partner pick the movie that you could care less about but they are stoked on. You might even learn that you love early '80s Steve Martin films.

Our brains are wired for us to be impacted by and dependent on one another. It is an oversimplification to say we are solely responsible for our emotions and needs. We all arrive at relationships with different strengths, challenges, and levels of privilege. We should aim for equity, in which all people in the relationship are encouraged to make requests and have opportunities for their needs to be met. As you look back on what you've now learned about your own relationship values and needs, how do they fit with ENM? Are the benefits of ENM worth facing your insecurities, fears, and feelings of discomfort?

PART II

How to Ethically Open Up

At this point, we are going to shift gears from asking whether ENM is a good fit for you to exploring how to navigate this relationship style effectively. Together we will look at some practical tips and suggestions for how to live out your values through practicing ENM. This will include making arrangements with partners, recognizing and responding to difficult emotions, and exercising communication skills.

It's understandable if you still have concerns. Even if you were to read every book there is on ENM, it is still likely that you will face obstacles and challenges at some point. Navigating a relationship style that is different from the social norm does have its complications. Change and transitions, as exciting as they can be, are hard. This section may impact your decision to change your approach to relationships, from subtle tweaks to a full overhaul. Shifting dynamics in relationships can feel particularly difficult because they shake up a sense of stability and can bring up fears for you or your partners, such as: *Will my partner meet someone they would rather be with than me? Will this person be better in bed than I am? What if I realize that I don't like this arrangement, but my partner does?* As you answer these questions, new ones will appear. I encourage you to approach ENM with curiosity, openness, and compassion. Regardless of the outcome, I am certain that through asking yourself these questions, you are opening yourself up to deeper and more fulfilling relationships.

4

Transforming Your Life

It is true that ENM can demand more effort than a monogamous relationship, simply because there are more people to care for. The best analogy I ever heard for this compared polyamory to owning houseplants. Some people choose to have one houseplant at a time because they feel sufficiently happy devoting their full attention and love toward it, and more than one plant would be too overwhelming. Other people find joy in filling their house with plants. They drape vines over their bookshelves, stack succulents on countertops, and hang ferns from the ceiling. Yes, it is more effort. In fact, they have to keep a schedule to remember to water, fertilize, and prune their green babies, but houseplants bring them so much joy that it is worth the extra effort. Imagine this section to be like reading a book titled *How to Keep My Plants Alive* and deciding if the effort is worth the outcome.

Being a Single Slut

Being single and ethically non-monogamous can take a variety of shapes. For some, it is a transition period between relationships and for others, it is a long-term lifestyle choice. There are a variety of ways to be a single slut, but some examples include: dating with the goal of finding relationships, dating with no intention of finding relationships, dating a couple as a **secondary partner**, and having multiple partners but living separately from them.

As we've touched on previously, our culture portrays singlehood as less desirable than being in a relationship. This can cloud our perceptions of what being single can look like and can make it seem that it isn't a perfectly acceptable life choice. It is important to validate being single as an option, not only for those who know this is a great fit for them, but also to help people who desire partnership to consciously choose this option rather than desperately clinging to a relationship out of fear that they are less-than without it.

What if you were to imagine choosing to be single—not as a backup plan or consolation prize, but because that would allow you to live your most ideal life? What would that look like? It may leave more opportunities to design a life on your terms without compromise. Perhaps more opportunities to travel, creating deep friendship bonds, taking risks at work, exploring creative projects, and being able to experience the passion and thrill in new connections.

Although loneliness is an increased risk in a single lifestyle, living unattached to a romantic partner also opens up the possibility of creating a community of deep connections.

There are drawbacks and challenges, of course, to a single lifestyle. For one, because our society tends to look down upon being single, there can be a stigma associated with it. If a person is dating someone in a couple, sometimes there can be poor treatment of the single one, particularly if the couple is new to ENM or underinformed. Take a look at the demeaning language that can be used to describe the single person: *homewrecker, secondary, the other woman.* Another challenge of being single is that you have to work more intentionally to cultivate a support system around you. It isn't a given who will be your emergency contact, wedding date, or vacation buddy. Although loneliness is an increased risk in a single lifestyle, living unattached to a romantic partner also opens up the possibility of creating a community of deep connections.

Joining a Triad/Throuple

If you decide to join an existing couple, there are some important questions to consider. It is necessary to have open communication with all the people involved and spend significant time talking about everyone's expectations, concerns, and boundaries. In comparison to a casual threesome, which necessitates only a conversation about consent, becoming a **throuple** requires a lot of thought and discussion beforehand. The lines of communication need to remain open throughout the relationship and, especially if it is your first time dating a pair, there are some challenges you might realize only over time. It can sometimes feel intimidating to bring up issues to the couple because they've been a team for longer, but remind yourself that if these partners are a good fit for you, they will want to help meet your needs.

In entering into an existing couple, it is typical that you will be taken on as their **third**. Consider how you feel about this positioning. Would you prefer to be in a more equal triad? What changes would need to be made in the relationship to help you feel more secure? Would this be a closed arrangement, or is it open to new partners? Are you able to continue dating while in this relationship? Reflect on your emotional and physical connection with both partners, as well as your personal boundaries. How compatible do you consider yourself to be with each partner?

Talk about what agreements or rules you have together as a throuple. Think over how you would like to distribute your time together. Will you have time with each partner individually or only as a unit? This is where starting a digital calendar together can streamline things. What are the expectations around openness with family, friends, and being in public together? Hopefully our society is becoming more accepting; as things stand, however, thirds are often not able to be included in family celebrations or work events. Check in with yourself if it would be too hard to see a photo on Instagram of your partners celebrating New Year's Eve with family while you're sitting at home.

Opening Up a Monogamous Relationship

Because it is the norm, many people fall into monogamy without giving it much thought. This means that a lot can be assumed without ever being explicitly communicated. Approach conversations about the structure of your relationship with the goal of bringing light to what has been unspoken. Monogamy may have worked really well in your relationship in the past—perhaps it provided a chance to build deep intimacy, trust, and security between the two of you alone—and it is now time for your relationship to shift and expand. It is okay if monogamy isn't working for you anymore. ENM is an exciting opportunity to express your needs and potentially grow with your partner.

Whether you've talked about opening your relationship together in the past but never specifically considered how to make it work, or this is your first time broaching the subject, it is okay to feel nervous. It is a vulnerable topic. It is helpful to keep in mind that this isn't a one-and-done conversation; everything does not need to be sorted out at once. In fact, it is helpful if you're able to take time to process everything being discussed. The conversation might bring up strong feelings, and someone's initial reaction to this discussion may not be where they land with it eventually. The beautiful thing about moving away from the monogamy script is that you are freeing each other up to design a relationship on your own terms. There are no set rules for how to open your relationship, and every relationship will have different needs and practices.

If your partner is brand-new to the concept of ENM, feel free to borrow a metaphor I heard at a party recently. A friend of mine explained the concept of ENM using cheese (they were speaking my language). I had shared with the group that I was working on a book about non-monogamy, and I was fielding some of the usual responses, including: *Oh I'd feel too insecure for that, I'd be super jealous, I'd worry my partner would leave.* Then my friend picked up the cheese plate and asked the group what their favorite cheese was.

Someone answered, "Gruyère."

My friend asked this person, "Is that the only cheese you like?"

"Oh no! I couldn't live without Grey Owl, Brie, or Gorgonzola."

"Does your love of Gorgonzola diminish the love you feel for Gruyère?"

"Oooh," went the room.

In early discussions with your partner about ENM, it is important to get clear on your *why* for opening things up. Is it for sex, relationships, or both? Also, will you be dating separately or as a couple? If you are dating separately, how much do you want to know about your partner's relationships? Consider whether knowing more or less information leads you to feel more secure in your relationship.

> ***Understand that the boundaries you set should be a living entity that you can continue to address through open communication.***

Because opening up relationships is a new endeavor, it is going to be a growing process. Understand that the boundaries you set should be a living entity that you can continue to address through open communication. You might begin this process not wanting any information about what your partner is doing (this is called a **Don't Ask Don't Tell**, or **DADT** situation) and find that this lack of information makes you feel too anxious. You might be surprised to learn that being able to ask your partner questions gives you a sense of ease. Part of the extra

PREEXISTING CONDITIONS

You already have a leg up on the process of opening your relationship if your connection with your partner is built on a foundation of trust, goodwill, mutual support, and clear communication. It's okay if you fight occasionally, because fighting in relationships is healthy and normal; what's important is that you fight fairly and fight friendly (which might sound like an oxymoron). This means you prioritize the love you have for each other over being right, go after the issue and not each other, avoid yelling, and express curiosity rather than defensiveness. Being able to handle conflict well puts you in the position to successfully navigate some of the challenging topics that will inevitably come up as you open your relationship.

Couples who have normalized talking about sexual and relationship needs and spent time examining how they want to structure their relationship together will find broaching this topic to be less emotionally charged. Although it may go without saying that it is easier to open up a relationship if both partners are keen on the idea, couples frequently differ on their level of interest. Many times with the clients I speak to in therapy, one partner is the advocate for opening the relationship, and the other is doing their best to go along with the idea. These couples can often still arrive at a healthy ENM relationship; however, the couples who transition most smoothly to non-monogamy are those in which both people are fully on the same page.

work of ENM is leaving a lot of space for processing feelings. Approach fears and feelings with curiosity, empathy, and openness. Think of this processing time like fertilizer for your houseplants: it might cost you a bit more time and effort, but the results will allow your relationship to thrive.

Are We Ready?

If you're considering opening up your monogamous relationship, I encourage you to sit down with your sweetie and discuss the following questions:

1. Why are we changing the structure of our relationship now?

2. What are you most excited about?

3. What are you afraid of?

4. What approach to ENM appeals to you— additional romantic partners, one-night stands, sex as a couple with others, sex with others separately?

5. If we want to be in a primary relationship together, what does that involve?

6. How much do you want to know about what the other person is doing? How do we know it is a good time to talk about this topic together? How often do we want to update each other on our behavior and relationships?

7. What kind of relationship do we want to have with each other's partners?

8. Are there certain people who are off-limits? Or certain places?

9. How will we come back together to reconnect after someone has been on a date?

10. What do you need to feel a little more secure with this new arrangement?

KEN AND JAMAL EXPLORE
OPENING UP

Ken (pronouns: he/him) and Jamal (pronouns: he/him) were struggling to connect sexually. In therapy, they learned to schedule a weekly *intimacy date*, where after they put the kids to bed, they made sure to spend some time together connecting in the bedroom. There was no pressure or expectation of sex; the goal was simply to be present with each other and engage in touch that felt good. This weekly ritual began to open up more space for sex and sensuality in their lives, and they began to incorporate discussing fantasies together.

A recurring theme that emerged through their fantasy sharing was an interest in exploring sex with new partners. Jamal began to realize it was something he actually wanted to try. He decided to initiate the conversation during a therapy session. He said, "Ken, I've noticed we've both shared that we would find it sexy to sleep with new people. I've been thinking that this might actually be something that would be fun to try out. I'm wondering where you sit with this?" At first, Ken said he felt surprised, and shared that he was interested, but he was worried it might be too emotionally difficult.

Through therapy, we began to focus on exploring their interests and concerns in opening their relationship, and after about six months they felt like they were ready to take the plunge. There were ups and downs in navigating which particular boundaries they found worked best for them, but eventually they found that they were able to finish therapy and continue practicing ENM together. They both felt they had the tools to communicate well and support each other, and they found meaning in the connections they were making. Ken and Jamal were also pleasantly surprised to find out that opening their relationship increased their sexual desire for one another.

When Not to Open Up

If you have one houseplant and it is dying, buying more houseplants isn't going to resurrect your decrepit fern. This is also the case with relationships. Adding more people to an already struggling relationship is just going to lead to more complications. It also isn't fair to bring other people into a dysfunctional relationship dynamic. Opening up your relationship should be a decision that is made when both partners are feeling loved, secure, and able to communicate effectively. If you've only ever been in monogamous relationships, consider how it can often cause trouble to enter into a rebound relationship too quickly after a breakup. If you haven't had sufficient time to regroup, process, and heal, you will inevitably dump baggage into the next relationship.

Opening up your relationship should be a decision that is made when both partners are feeling loved, secure, and able to communicate effectively.

Take stock of your existing relationship, including the capacity you and your partner have to regulate your emotions. Are you happy in your current relationship? Do you generally have warm feelings toward your partner and feel sexually satisfied? If the answer is no, it is important to reflect on your reasoning behind why you are considering this decision. Be particularly wary of deciding to open up a relationship after an infidelity. Opening up a relationship after someone has cheated can be very tempting as a Band-Aid solution. It is almost saying: "There! Now this isn't a breach of trust anymore." But it *was* a breach of trust, and infidelity in a relationship can often cause a huge rupture that needs time to repair. The process of opening up requires the relationship to be already built on a solid foundation of trust. There will be challenging conversations and tricky circumstances to navigate, particularly at the beginning, and both people need to feel comfortable turning toward each other to work through these moments together.

Mono/Poly Relationships

It's not uncommon for monogamous folks to hitch up with polyamorous people. As the term highlights, a **mono/poly** relationship is one in which one partner is monogamous and the other is polyamorous. For many, the decision to be monogamous or polyamorous represents one of their foundational guiding beliefs. The conflicts that can come with this divide are not unlike those of couples who have differing religious beliefs: there may be a friction of perspectives on anything from the role of extended family to the meaning of life. Although there are certainly ways to work around differences with both religious beliefs and approaches to monogamy, it's important to emphasize that it can be a challenging arrangement.

If you are in a mono/poly arrangement, you must love and accept your partner for who they are now.

To successfully navigate these differences, both partners must first recognize that they are entering into a situation that requires extra self-awareness, emotional intelligence, communication, and, frankly, effort. Both partners must determine what their core relationship values and needs are, and check that they will not be put in a position to compromise them frequently or for too long. Just as you would if your partner had different religious beliefs, it is paramount that you respect what leads them to feel fulfilled. The mono/poly couple also needs to be wary of falling in love with potential, meaning that they are expecting or anticipating that the other partner will eventually change their beliefs. This only leads to hurt and resentment. If you are in a mono/poly arrangement, you must love and accept your partner for who they are now.

Strategies for the Mono Partner

It is inevitable, if you are the monogamous partner, that at some point you will experience uncomfortable emotions. Start by naming the feeling, and know that whatever emotion comes up is okay. Having hard feelings doesn't mean that you have failed or that you're unable to function in this relationship. Have compassion for yourself and the fact that you're choosing a more challenging path. There will be struggle, but there will also be growth. If, for you, the value of the relationship outweighs the struggle, carry on.

Remind yourself that your partner's polyamorous identity has nothing to do with you. It is about them living fully in their values. Nothing about you would change this—not your attractiveness, your sexual capabilities, or your intelligence. As you are now, you are enough. Love in healthy relationships is not earned; it is given freely and in abundance. Know that it is okay to ask for help. Practice asking for what you need from your partner (we will touch on how to communicate this in chapter 6). Remind yourself of the benefits of the mono/poly arrangement. For example, it takes the pressure off you to try to be everything for your partner, which may allow more space in your life to pursue other interests and hobbies. It is also an opportunity to devote more energy to deepening your friendships. Being with a polyamorous person also gives you the beautiful experience of your partner choosing you repeatedly—not out of obligation, but because they want to.

Strategies for the Poly Partner

If you are the polyamorous partner, check in with the reasons ENM is important to you. Is this a decision you're making to more closely align with your values, such as freedom, openness to experiences, and making new connections? Dig deep and be wary if your reasons are to try to fix a strained relationship or to buffer yourself until you find a new partner. If you know you're being fully honest with yourself and your partner, know that your needs are completely valid. It is wonderful that you are listening to yourself and recognizing what is important for you in relationships.

Understand that asking your monogamous partner to buck cultural norms around relationships has its difficulties. Have patience and leave space for your partner's emotions as they make this transition. Your partner may also require some extra reassurance of your love and commitment to the relationship from time to time. Consider what your nonnegotiable needs and boundaries are within the relationship and be willing to be flexible to meet your partner's needs outside of those. For example, it may be essential to your need for freedom to spend weekends away with your other partners, but you may be willing to call your primary partner on the phone each day that you are apart.

Setting Boundaries

Personal boundaries refer to what you will and will not tolerate from others. You have physical boundaries around what type of touch you will tolerate where on your body and from whom, and you also have psychological boundaries, which is your metaphorical skin that protects your mind and emotions from the behavior or ideologies (e.g., racism, sexism, homophobia) of others. Only you can determine your boundaries. It can feel quite scary and vulnerable to set your boundaries within relationships because they are tied to your personal values, needs, and fears.

Setting boundaries with others is about communicating your no-go zones, the behavior you will not tolerate under any circumstances. Maintaining boundaries is not an attempt to control your partner or an effort to create certainty in the relationship. Both efforts, of course, would be futile. Boundary-setting is often more challenging than it sounds, because in moments of discomfort in relationships, it is tempting to jump to setting a strict rule to feel like you have more control over a situation.

Imagine holding a butterfly in your outstretched hand. The butterfly represents your relationship, and your hand is your personal boundary. The trust you build in your relationship is beautiful and delicate; it involves the support of your palm. If you discover that the butterfly is poisonous, you would understandably brush it off your hand because you wouldn't choose to get hurt for the benefit of the insect. However, if you were to become so fearful that the butterfly

Boundary Questions

You will know if your boundary has been crossed because it will elicit a visceral response. It could be anything from a physical tightness to an increased heart rate or dizziness. You may also feel it emotionally as bitterness, nervousness, frustration, anger, exhaustion, or shame. When you tune in to your body responses and emotions, it will get easier to express your relationship needs, desires, and boundaries. I encourage you to leave a few moments after each questions to notice how your body responds.

1. What's a time in the past when I felt like a boundary was crossed? How did I know? What did my body feel like? What emotions did it bring up?

2. What does it feel like when my boundaries are respected? What does my body feel like? What emotions get brought up?

3. What's a boundary I'm not honoring in my own life right now, perhaps with friends, coworkers, or family?

4. What do I need to feel a little more secure in my relationship?

5. What feelings come up when I consider expressing boundaries in my relationship?

We are just skimming the surface on the topic of boundaries here. For more in-depth work, I recommend checking out the Resources section (page 177).

would fly away that you curl your fingers tightly, you might unintentionally crush its wings. If your relationship is based in fear, it will never experience real trust.

When you communicate your boundaries to your partner/s, try to identify the need underneath the feeling that is coming up. For example, if you notice you feel worried when your partner is not home, a fear-based response may be to ask them to have a curfew. But, maybe, underneath this worry, your need is for reassurance, security, or predictability. There are usually a variety of ways to have a need met, so perhaps a way to support you with this is for your partner to send you a text check-in, to give you 24 hours' notice before a date, or to provide a pre-written note of their commitment to you that you can read in moments of stress.

Establishing Agreements

Most of us get by in our day-to-day lives with our relationships following the implied social norms. We know to shake hands when we meet someone new at work, to offer to help clean up after a dinner party, and to tip the server after a meal. We become so used to these unspoken expectations that it can be jarring when faced with a different set of norms (like if you've ever been greeted with a kiss on both cheeks). Just because we've gotten used to one way of doing things doesn't mean it is the best way. Creating agreements in your relationship/s is a wonderful way to make explicit what is implicit so you can decide what works best for you and your partner. Particularly in ENM relationships, it is helpful to establish agreements that work for your particular relationship because there isn't a set of social norms to follow.

When I first moved in with my partner, I was incredibly nervous. It felt like a giant step, and I was worried about entering this unknown territory. My therapist encouraged me to make a list of agreements with my partner. At first I thought this was an unnecessary and cheesy suggestion. *Really?* I thought. *Do you want me to put that right beside my vision board?* But I decided to give it a try, and it ended up being an incredibly helpful practice and opened up some important conversations in my relationship. The agreement included everything from how we would divide housework to what we considered cheating, as well as how we intend to respond if someone does cheat. Not only was the discussion of the agreements valuable, but so was the suggestion of writing them down. Having a tangible copy allows for accountability and clarity, as well as tangible evidence for how relationship agreements can change over time.

When I introduce the concept of setting agreements to my clients, people respond either with eagerness or a thinly veiled eye roll. I can understand the resistance because I reacted that way, too. I think our resistance to setting agreements can often be another iteration of the classic trap that people fall into in their relationships: We expect our partners to be able to read our minds. If they are unable to do so, we attribute this to an incompatibility in the relationship. As a result, it is considered romantic blasphemy to write down what it is we need to feel happier and more secure in relationships. The truth is, of course, that we are not relational mediums, so being open to having these discussions with our partners can be incredibly beneficial.

When you first make relationship agreements, know that they do not have to be perfectly articulated and that they are not set in stone. Particularly if non-monogamy is a new structure to your relationship, you couldn't possibly anticipate each agreement that would benefit you. If you begin to wonder whether you are following an agreement, that is a sign to get more specific together. If you notice that you continually have a sense of unease or discomfort in your relationship, that also might mean there is a need for a new agreement. Any partner can request to discuss a change at any time; the agreements simply provide the framework for you and your partner/s to become better aligned within the relationship. In ENM relationships, it can be particularly helpful to create agreements around the topics in the following sections.

Planning Time and Scheduling

A key element to successfully maneuvering multiple relationships is to be thoughtful about how you organize your time with your partners. If you are in a non-hierarchical polyamorous relationship, it can be a balancing act that ebbs and flows. Clear communication is necessary, and the use of a shared calendar is highly recommended.

It is helpful to consider what you need to manage feelings of discomfort around your partner dating other people. Some couples have an ongoing practice of finding time together to talk and connect and share feelings before or soon after one of them goes on a date. Others may have more straightforward requests, such as to split the fee for a babysitter or not to text or have phone conversations with other partners in front of each other.

Many people find that creating some form of predictability for when their partner will go on a date helps manage the feelings of anxiety that can arise. This predictability can look like asking their partner to tell them in advance before they go on a date. Whether it is a day or a week in advance, this notice provides the person with the opportunity to make alternative plans to deal with the stress (remember Billie's platonic sleepover from chapter 3?), as well as to mentally prepare. For people who feel that planning tramples on the free and fun aspect of ENM, I invite you to consider a compromise and arrange certain days of the calendar or trips where you can be sexually spontaneous. This compromise works to create predictability for the unpredictability.

Hierarchy; Primary/Secondary Poly

All people in the relationship, whether they are considered to be a primary or a secondary partner, have the right to be treated with respect, communicate their needs, and have opportunities to have these needs met. Keep all partners in mind when making agreements, whether it's an open or polyamorous arrangement. Acknowledge how power is distributed and take extra care to extend compassion and respect to secondary partners, who are often forgotten about in the agreement process. Secondary partners are fully entitled to articulate boundaries and request agreements.

All people in the relationship, whether they are considered to be a primary or a secondary partner, have the right to be treated with respect, communicate their needs, and have opportunities to have these needs met.

If you are a couple who is looking to open your relationship, keep the lines of communication open about whether you are making this decision for the purpose of novel sexual connections or a multitude of relationships. It's okay if your ENM desires change over time; what matters is that you are truthful about your intentions with your partner/s. Couples in open relationships may have agreements around telling their partner if they have an emotional or sexual connection that impacts their relationship, as well as telling all new partners that they are in a committed primary relationship.

Anonymous Sex

Some couples who open their relationship may feel more comfortable with the idea of only having sex with people they will never see again. These couples might feel that there is less threat to the existing relationship if there are only opportunities for one-time sexual encounters. This may look like sexual experiences together at play parties, in BDSM dungeons, or in threesomes. Or, it could look like permission for each partner to sleep with other people separately for one-off experiences. This may be with someone they meet online, at a bar, or while traveling for work. For safety reasons, if someone in the couple is meeting up with a new date, it might be in their relationship agreement to let their partner know where they will be and to be reachable by phone.

Some couples also chose to have a **DADT** relationship in which no details are shared about their sexual experiences with other people. In my therapy practice, I often see that people are drawn to this relationship structure when they are new to non-monogamy; over time, however, it often leads to heightened anxiety and lowered trust. If you fall into this category, I would encourage you to get curious with yourself about what it is about anonymity or withholding information that leads you to feel more comfortable. This may be a sign of internalized sex-negativity and shame, or a desire to avoid potentially uncomfortable feelings. All this can be rich content to reflect on and process.

Vetoes

Whether to have veto rights is a controversial issue within ENM circles. If there is veto power in the relationship, it means that one person can make the decision to ask their partner to stop dating someone. Many believe that vetoes are manipulative and compromise freedom in the relationship. Others believe that vetoes are simply another articulation of a personal boundary. Although a veto can be issued like a command to end a relationship with one specific person, the people in the relationship can also decide together what types of people are off-limits for dating. These individuals can include coworkers, classmates, close friends, ex-partners, neighbors, relatives, and so on.

To implement a veto effectively and fairly, it is necessary to speak from your own perspective and make a request, rather than issue a command. This piece is just like communicating healthy boundaries. We will continue to practice speaking from the "I" perspective in chapter 6. Before a veto is enacted, you need to hear your partner's input and consent. For example, say, "When you date your ex, it makes me feel insecure and worried. I'm wondering if you'd consider ending your sexual relationship." Rather than, "You need to stop seeing her."

Conflict Resolution

As hard as we might try, as humans, it is not possible to be free of conflict or disagreement with others. We encounter areas of disagreement all the time in our relationships with our families, friends, and coworkers. However, when it comes to our romantic and sexual relationships, it can feel daunting to have opposing viewpoints from the person so intimately intertwined in your life.

DANA AND LUIS

Dana (pronouns: she/her) and Luis (pronouns: he/him) initially came to counseling for tools to help with Luis's erectile dysfunction. The couple spoke about how over the past year, when they attempted to have sex, they would end up in a big fight. When Dana felt that it was taking Luis too long to get an erection, she would get exasperated and make a sweeping statement like, "We'll never have a normal sex life!" Luis would shut down, which would leave Dana feeling even more frustrated until she would finally go to another room.

What helped this couple was to get vulnerable rather than defensive with each other, and to communicate compassionately. Dana was eventually able to express that in those moments she felt worried that she wasn't as attractive as Luis's other partners and thought his silence meant he didn't care about her. Luis was able to communicate that he loved her so much that he felt buried in shame not to be able to satisfy her sexually. The couple realized what they both needed in those moments was to make sex less stressful and to find a way to connect with each other rather than put up walls. As Dana and Luis improved their communication with each other, they began to be able to identify their unhelpful pattern earlier. They started broadening how they defined sex to take the pressure off penetration and emphasized pleasure and connection.

You may differ with your partner on what your preferred approach to non-monogamy is, how often you'd like to talk on the phone, or your favorite sexual position. When making agreements together, there will likely be the need for some compromise. Consider where you are not willing to bend because doing so would significantly impact your sense of happiness and security. It is helpful to consider the question, *Where are you willing to give in the relationship in exchange for what you get in return?* Sex advice columnist Dan Savage refers to this as the **price of admission**. For example, if your metamour does not like you, is this a price of admission you're willing to pay to be with your partner?

It is best to speak about a conflict when neither you nor your partner is feeling heightened emotions. Sometimes this means taking a pause together to take a few breaths, taking a 20-minute time-out, or tabling an issue for a later date. If you are in the middle of an argument, it can be helpful to practice communicating to each other to take a pause. Noticing when you are falling into unhelpful patterns takes practice, and I encourage you to come up with a code word or a hand signal when one of you notices this pattern; the word or hand signal for *time-out* works great, but *cartwheel, snickerdoodle,* or *sassafras* does the trick, too (I think the sillier the code word the better, because how can you keep fighting after saying *snickerdoodle?*).

Remember that the strongest relationships believe in repairs; they do not live in fear of ruptures.

If you are taking a pause, setting a particular time limit is helpful so you are both aware that you will revisit the topic. When you approach the topic again from a more grounded place, allow each person their space to talk. Speak from your own perspective and avoid blaming the other person. Extend empathy, nonjudgment, and goodwill to your partner. Remember that the love in your relationship is more important than being right. Make small concessions with each other that do not compromise your boundaries. For example, you may not be able to find 50-50 agreement, but sometimes an 80-20 agreement will be a workable solution for both of you. Conflict in relationships is healthy and normal. Remember that the strongest relationships believe in repairs; they do not live in fear of ruptures.

HOOKUP AND DATING APPS

In many ways, the use of dating apps has simplified the process of meeting partners as an ENM person. With dating apps in general, one of the nice things is that you can be completely upfront about who you are and what you're looking for without having to "come out" to people over and over again. Whether you're non-monogamous, kinky, or STI-positive, or have a physical impairment or diagnosis, you can put it all out there. This way people can screen themselves, and you don't have to waste any time with someone who won't be a fit for you.

Using apps can get tricky if you have concerns about confidentiality. It is a particularly sticky issue if partners in a couple have different needs around being "out." Some people may simply be uncomfortable with being "out," and others could risk serious ramifications to employment or family life. If you find yourself in a conflict about being "out" through dating apps, it is helpful to visit the conversation of what non-monogamy means for you in general and in your relationship. Are you simply looking for playmates in the bedroom? Are you looking for something more akin to polyamory? Or perhaps something in between. Our sex lives are generally private, so it's understandable to want to keep this part of your life separate. You may not want a coworker to know you're swinging because a friend of a friend saw you on Hinge. On the other hand, if you're looking to begin partnerships, I encourage you to seriously consider where you can be open about this part of your life; it is degrading and hurtful to treat one of your partners as a sexual secret rather than a relationship.

Meeting Other People

If you're feeling ready to date non-monogamously, you may be wondering about where to begin meeting people. Many single monogamous people worry about finding potential partners, so it is understandable for people keen on ENM to also worry about where they will find partners. The good news is that, in many ways, dating as a non-monogamous person is very similar to dating as a monogamous person.

If you are looking to begin dating as a polyamorous person, it is possible that you may meet someone you are interested in during your everyday life; it is less likely, however, that they will also identify as non-monogamous. If you decide to begin dating someone and you are unsure about their stance on non-monogamy, it is important to tell them as early as you feel comfortable. If you are dating online, it can be beneficial to put your interest in non-monogamy on your profile or to text the person before your first date.

It can streamline your search for a partner to look specifically for people who openly identify as polyamorous or non-monogamous. One of the most popular dating sites among polyamorous people is OkCupid because it provides poly options on the profile and search queries. It is also helpful to begin expanding your social circle of non-monogamous friends. Most cities have Meetup and Facebook groups where you can chat with people both online and in person. Make sure to read the group guidelines because many groups specifically prohibit asking people on dates in the group or at particular events. This is a great policy to help people feel free to connect without stress. If this policy feels frustrating, understand that it is important not to make every social event about meeting a partner because this can put a lot of pressure on you, which in turn makes it more challenging to form authentic connections. Recognize the value of gaining more non-monogamous friends who can understand and support your experiences. And hey, by creating genuine friendships, you're also organically expanding opportunities to meet friends of friends who may be poly.

Right to Privacy

It is a personal choice whether to be out to others about your poly-amorous or non-monogamous identity. There are benefits and risks to both options. If you choose to be fully open about your relationships, you are able to live your life free of the burden of hiding your authentic self. You will know that the people in your life accept you for who you are. You are also more likely to be able to find potential partners. There is also, unfortunately, the threat of judgment from others and the stresses that come from living a life outside of what's socially expected. Keeping your non-monogamous identity private does buffer you from the social stigma, but it forces you to hide core elements of yourself.

Another risk to keeping your polyamorous relationship secret is that it leaves you more vulnerable to being trapped in an abusive dynamic. One of the most common tactics an abuser will use is to cut someone off from their family and friends. If you do not feel you have anyone you can speak to about your relationship, there are fewer opportunities for someone to validate your experiences and spot if you are being mistreated. Outside of an abusive situation, it is still incredibly valuable to have a support system where you can talk honestly about your relationship. Having other polyamorous people for support is ideal because you can get advice and hear other people's experiences beyond just your partner. If it is not possible for you to be open about your non-monogamous identity right now, that is completely okay. Reflect on where you may be able to speak about your relationship, whether with a select few trusted friends or through an online support group.

Sharing Your Relationships with the World

I am hopeful that our culture is moving in a direction that is more accepting of the variety of ways people choose to love and live their lives that are not harmful to others. At this time, however, there are still risks to being out as an ENM person. People can get fired, lose emotional and financial support from family, have custody of their children taken away, and be punished by dishonorable discharge from the military. There is a certain amount of privilege afforded to people who are able to come out to the world as polyamorous without any risk.

We have many rituals in our culture that flaunt monogamy: engagement rings, weddings, and Instagram posts about anniversaries are all a public declaration of one type of relationship. Prejudice is based in ignorance, and the more people realize ENM is all around them, the more the stigma will lift. Consider how societal acceptance of BDSM increased after the popularization of the *Fifty Shades of Grey* saga (a terrible depiction of BDSM, but that's a topic for another book). Or, as more people proclaim their queer identities, the more others are able to as well. Campaigns such as Dan Savage's It Gets Better Project understand the power of visibility, with more than 70,000 LGBTQ+ people sharing their own stories to help queer youth feel less alone. We see the same rates of people practicing consensual non-monogamy regardless of factors such as race, religion, age, income, education level, or political affiliation. Although some may argue that how they choose to live their life is no one else's business, it is undeniable that the more people publicly claim polyamorous identities, the more others will feel safe to do the same.

You Can Start Here

If you are feeling like you want to share your non-monogamous or polyamorous identity with the world, it can feel daunting to know where to start.

1. Remember that your sexual identity is valid. Monogamy doesn't determine morality. As long as you are treating others with kindness and respect, you get to decide who you love and who to have sex with. Even if someone responds with judgment, you have nothing to be ashamed of.

2. Know that there is no right or wrong way to share this information. Consider what makes you feel the most comfortable, whether it is in person, through text, or over the phone. Does this person tend to respond better when they have time to digest the information? Send a text. Or, do you personally want to be there to hear their reaction? Tell them in person, or give them a call if you need a quick exit strategy.

3. Offer some introductory information about what polyamory is. (There are some excellent options in the Resources, page 177.)

4. Use your boundaries. Know what you are and are not willing to hold space for. You may be willing to answer some basic questions, but end the conversation if you feel they are dumping their fear onto you.

5. Point them in the direction of where to learn more. This may be new information to the people you are telling, and they may need some time to process. That does not mean it is your responsibility to teach them. If you do not have the emotional capacity to walk them through things, you can certainly point them in the direction of some introductory books, like *Opening Up*, *The Ethical Slut*, or even the book in your hands!

5

Recognizing Jealousy and Other Hard Feelings

A common hesitation toward non-monogamy comes from a reluctance to feel difficult emotions like jealousy, shame, and rejection. Ethically non-monogamous folks invite these challenging experiences through the front door, not out of masochism but from an understanding that we are meant to experience *all* the emotions, even the painful ones. Our feelings carry information and opportunities for growth and deepened connection. The choices we make for our lives should be in pursuit of our values, not in avoidance of potential hurt.

If I could boil down the process of therapy to a simple phrase, it would be *It's okay to feel the hard feelings*. It can be incredibly valuable to build your emotional vocabulary. Having the language to describe your emotions in detail and understand the needs associated with them strengthens your connection with yourself and with others.

To enhance your emotional literacy, I encourage you to google a list of emotions or a "Feelings Wheel." Keep the list nearby or on your phone and consult it to help you identify your emotional state at various points throughout the day. Some people find it helpful to keep a journal to specifically identify and record their emotions.

Emotional Honesty and Resilience

We can't pick and choose which feelings we want to feel. Even as a therapist, where it is in my job description to work with and understand emotions, this seems to be a lesson I need to learn again and again. When we try to suppress emotions like anger or sadness, we also end up preventing ourselves from experiencing feelings like joy and ease. Emotions have a beginning, a middle, and an end. We need to let them wash over us to get to the other side.

All emotions are information, and there is nothing wrong with any emotion we feel at any time. Where we get into trouble is how we respond to our emotions. As a kid, I sometimes watched *The Oprah Winfrey Show* after school. On one episode, Oprah talked to Dr. Oz about gas. I remember my 12-year-old mind was blown when Oprah advocated on national television for people not to hold in their farts. What do farts have to do with our emotions? Buckle up, we're going for a fart metaphor. Our emotions are like gas: Some people find this natural bodily function so inexcusable that they will do whatever they can to suppress it, and if it sneaks out, they hope to god no one ever notices. Others proactively deny or blame, making their emotions someone else's problem. And though, just as Dr. Oz said, "be smart about it, do it in a place that's airy enough that you're not going to hurt your family and friends," we also want to be conscious of where and when we find our emotional release. Our feelings, like flatulence, need to move through us. Once they are felt, they will pass.

Recognizing Jealousy

Jealousy is a feeling that, if given the choice, many of us would click "unsubscribe." This emotion can be understood as a feeling that arises when you believe something of yours is being threatened. A subtle but helpful distinction: jealousy is different from envy. **Envy** is a feeling that pops up when we see someone else having something that we want. In considering these two emotions within relationships, jealousy involves the threat of the "third," which can be real (such as your partner's other partner), or perceived (such as a looming threat that your partner may one day cheat on you). Envy is just between you and someone else, meaning that you want something they have (such as an outfit, award, or vacation), but you are not worried it is a threat to any of your relationships.

Fortunately or unfortunately, jealousy is not something we can avoid as humans, regardless of our relationship structure. Jealousy is actually identifiable in infants as early as three months old. It makes sense that most pop psych texts on polyamory dedicate a significant amount of focus to managing jealousy, because it is a relationship structure where the people consciously choose to invite the "third" (real or abstract) into their lives every day.

While jealousy is usually uncomfortable, it can often feel unbearable. Clementine Morrigan, in their writing and teaching about the intersection of polyamory and trauma, speaks about moving away from using the word "jealousy" and instead using the term "distress." As we'll explore in chapter 7, people with attachment injuries and relational trauma can experience overwhelming reactions when they perceive their relationship security to be threatened. Jealousy can get fused with fear of abandonment, anger, shame, and other emotions that can be experienced intensely by the nervous system, eliciting a full fight, flight, or freeze response. "Distress" more accurately captures this reaction, which can look like anything from sweating to racing thoughts to scrolling endlessly on Instagram. A better understanding of the connection to the nervous system response also opens you up to more strategies to support yourself in moments of distress.

There is often a stigma around jealousy in mainstream polyamorous communities. I have frequently heard my poly clients worry that they have failed at being poly when they feel jealous. Self-criticism only fans the flames of the struggle. When you can understand the root of your jealousy and be with it without judgment, you will be able to look at your jealousy as a teacher—albeit a kind of thorny one.

When you can understand the root of your jealousy and be with it without judgment, you will be able to look at your jealousy as a teacher—albeit a kind of thorny one.

Jealousy Triggers

In our culture of compulsory monogamy, we get some toxic messages about the role of jealousy in love. Toxic monogamy messaging puts out the unrealistic pressure that not only will you be with one partner for the rest of your life, you will also always be the only priority in each other's lives, and if you or your partner even *considers* being attracted to anyone else, something is terribly wrong. Because the stakes feel so high, people can become hypervigilant, constantly looking for signs that their partner is cheating (and maybe taking a Louisville slugger to both headlights, à la Carrie Underwood). On top of this pressure, there is mixed messaging about the role of jealousy. It is positioned both as a personal failing for the person who experiences it and as a sign of love and worthiness if it's displayed by your partner.

I want to emphasize that jealousy is normal, *not* a moral failing. With that said, it is understandable, given the compulsory monogamy culture, that certain experiences trigger jealousy more readily than others. For example, because our society privileges the couple above other relationship formations, people may feel jealous if they believe their couple status is threatened. People in polyamorous relationships can also internalize compulsory monogamy messaging, and may feel jealous if they feel their partner is prioritizing their metamour. For example, jealousy may arise if someone's metamour gets to have a more public relationship with their partner than they do, whether through inclusion at family events, PDA, or posting together on social media.

Experiences of jealousy also intersect with experiences of gender. In our patriarchal society, the female message is that sexual desirability equals relationship stability, and the male message is that performance, whether financial, athletic, or sexual, is what's important. When these sources of self-worth are challenged, perhaps by observing your

What Makes Me Jealous?

In moments when we are hijacked by jealousy, it can be challenging to see it as an impermanent state. It is helpful to sit down and reflect on your own relationship fears and jealousy triggers when you are in a calm state of mind. This way, when you experience moments of jealousy, you will more easily be able to see the fearmongering script for what it is, and you will be more able to talk about it and let the moment wash over you.

1. How do I know when I am feeling jealous? What body sensations do I notice? What emotions feel strongest? What do my thought patterns look like?

2. Is there a metaphor that best describes my experience of jealousy? For example, it feels like I'm drowning, running but not getting anywhere, lost in the forest.

3. When was the most recent time I've noticed this response? Was I with a certain person? Have I felt this way around them before?

4. What do I judge most frequently in others?

5. What unmet need am I expressing through my judgment?

partner flirting with someone else, it can create jealousy rooted in the fear of not being good enough.

Another common trigger in polyamorous relationships can be when you are confronted with evidence of the sex your partner is

SURPRISED BY JEALOUSY

Of all the uncomfortable emotions, jealousy is a particularly gross one for me to feel. So much so that not too long ago I would have told you with a shrug that "I don't really get jealous anymore." I have come to learn that when we write off entire emotions, there's usually something fishy going on beneath our awareness.

A few years ago, I started to get curious about the intense judgmental thoughts I had when a particular Instagram account I followed posted sexy selfies. As someone who is sex-positive and a big supporter of women making their own choices about their bodies, I felt embarrassed that this woman's bikini photo collection was so enraging to me.

I started to ask myself, *What unmet need am I expressing through this judgment?* Then it dawned on me: *Oh shit, I'm jealous.* I had previously labeled jealousy as "bad" and had put it in the "do not feel" filing cabinet. I realized that this woman, about whom I knew very little, was bringing up my own unmet need to express my sensual side. I grew up in an environment where expressions of sexiness were explicitly criticized, and I was only then unearthing this formerly banished desire. In acknowledging the unmet need brought up by my jealousy, I was able to begin to allow more space in my life to engage this side of myself. When I gave myself permission to explore what sexy means to me, the judgment and jealousy stopped feeling so intense.

having with someone else. Whether it is a sext, a condom wrapper, or another partner's underwear, these experiences can send you into a jealous spiral even when you are okay with your arrangement on a rational level. This type of jealousy can also be evidence of old programming from our culture that teaches us that if your partner has sex with someone else, you have lost something. The good news is that by learning to identify your own jealousy triggers, you will be able to hold more compassion for yourself and allow the feeling to dissipate on its own without letting it hold too much weight.

Accepting Jealousy

No relationship style can safeguard you from jealousy. Because of how uncomfortable it can feel, it is possible that jealousy is an emotion you exiled long ago. Unfortunately, when we suppress emotions or criticize ourselves for having particular ones, we just give them more momentum to come up stronger. I wish there was a way to opt out of the terrible feeling of jealousy, but unfortunately there's not a whole lot you can do to be rid of it. Rather than fight with jealousy, I encourage you to turn toward it with calm curiosity.

When you first notice the prickly feeling of jealousy, take some deep breaths to let your body settle down. Because jealousy can so often be muddled with other emotions, such as guilt, fear, resentment, and so on, take a moment to identify what core emotions are coming up. Remind yourself that you are capable of feeling whatever is there, however uncomfortable it is, and that the sensation will not last forever. Identify the insecurity, longing, or unmet need underneath your emotional response. From there, be honest with your partner about how you're feeling and what you need—whether it's a nonjudgmental ear, validation, or a just a hug. Consider how a healthy relationship isn't based on the absence of jealousy, but the ability to speak openly about it.

Know that on the other side of jealousy, there is even the possibility for compersion, in which you find joy in your partner's joy; for example, being excited for your partner's new relationship energy (NRE). You've already got the capacity for this feeling of compersion—it's not much different from the warm, fuzzy feeling that arises spontaneously when watching people dance with abandon in the pride parade, a child laugh wildly, or puppies cuddling. Compersion and jealousy are not mutually exclusive, they are often present at the same time. In addition to identifying how jealousy shows up in your body, thoughts, and emotions, take some time to build a picture of what compersion feels like for you. When you have the language for this feeling, you will more easily be able to tap into it.

Recognizing Shame

The Shame Wizard is a character from the Netflix cartoon *Big Mouth*. Apart from being a hilarious show about puberty, the writers absolutely nail their personification of shame. The Shame Wizard appears suddenly to John Mulaney's character one day after he is caught masturbating. The wizard tells the young boy how he's "wretched" and "a loathsome little pervert," and that "he'll *never* feel better." From then on, the boy is haunted by shame, oscillating between feeling completely immobilized and lashing out in anger toward others. Later in the show, the Shame Wizard confesses that he actually doesn't have malevolent intent. In fact, he truly does want his haunting to help people better themselves to maintain social harmony.

There are a few reasons this character is a fantastic portrayal of shame. First, shame is a social emotion, so it typically originates in a social context. We often learn shame from others, whether from religion, the media, our parents, or peers. For some of my clients, they can pinpoint exact moments where they remembered learning shame, and for others it is the result of a cumulation of experiences.

Our shame stories typically form our negative core beliefs, which are deeply held ideas about ourselves, others, and the world. Common negative core beliefs rooted in shame include: "I'm too much," "I'm unlovable," "I'm abnormal," and "I'm stupid." Although shame starts in a social experience, we eventually internalize it, creating our very own Shame Wizard.

Shame also has good intentions; it wants us to stay connected to the group, and it's terrified if this tie becomes threatened. Despite its positive intentions, when we are buried in shame, we are not actually able to respond effectively. Here, a distinction between guilt and shame is beneficial. Shame is the belief that "I am bad," whereas guilt is the understanding that "I did something bad." With shame, we either internalize the experience and fall so deeply into a hole of self-condemnation that we become paralyzed, or we externalize it and lash out to others with anger. When we learn from our unhelpful behavior and make amends or respond more effectively in the future, it is guilt that is leading the charge.

Shame is a frequent symptom for survivors of physical, emotional, and sexual abuse. Shame can almost be worn as armor, an attempt to shape some certainty. It is an understandable reaction, because the experience of abuse is typically unpredictable and uncontrollable. If the survivor consciously or unconsciously determines there was something wrong with them, they may be able to find a way to change and prevent it from happening again.

Because of our sex-negative culture, shame infiltrates many people's relationships with sex. In my work as a sex therapist, many times with sexual dysfunctions, biology is not the problem; *shame* is the problem. Internalized messaging from our upbringing, or religion, or porn tells us that if we don't fit certain expectations, we are worthless. A lot of the healing work involves beginning to understand that their sexual desires are healthy and wonderful, and the idea of "normal" sexuality is a myth.

Compulsory monogamy in our society can also create shame triggers for people who are daring to live outside these expectations. Some toxic monogamy messaging includes a scarcity mindset around love, including that there is only *one* soul mate and that real love means monogamy. There is judgment that if your partner loves or wants to have sex with someone else, it's because something is wrong with you. Oof. Talk about shame material.

Challenging your negative core beliefs and speaking to yourself more kindly are fantastic ways to start unraveling a shame spiral. Because shame is a social emotion, the remedy is to receive compassion and empathy from others. That is why therapy can be so powerful, because it is a witnessing of experience without judgment. Writing

MO RECOGNIZES
MOUNTING SHAME

Mo (pronouns: she/her) noticed that a self-critical dialogue would run through her brain during sex. She was in an ENM relationship with her partner, Ted, and lately she observed that she was negatively comparing herself sexually to Ted's other partners. Mo would feel weighed down by shame, and as a result, she remained very quiet during sex. Ted would check in with her a few times to ask if she was okay. Eventually, Mo would blow up in anger and defensiveness. She would blame Ted and say something like, "How do you expect me to be comfortable when you're out fucking half the city?!" This would instigate a big argument, and they wouldn't speak to each other for a few days.

Mo began to realize the unhelpful pattern she was falling into, and how she was trying to avoid shame and vulnerability by channeling it into rage. One day she approached Ted and expressed what she was feeling under her anger. She told Ted, "This is really difficult for me to share, but I'm realizing that I'm experiencing a lot of insecurity in our relationship right now. I feel embarrassed because ENM is something I really want, and I wish this didn't feel so uncomfortable for me." Ted responded with a sigh of relief, "I had no idea you were feeling this way. You know you are so important to me for so many reasons and I also love having sex with you for many, *many* reasons." Mo also felt like a weight had been lifted and told Ted that just being able to express her insecurities was extremely helpful, and she also realized that verbal reassurance and compliments from Ted would help combat her feelings of shame.

Overcoming Shame

The antidote to shame is empathy and compassion. When shame has got you in a choke hold, I encourage you to reach out to speak with supportive people in your life, as well as to speak to yourself with kindness. Some of the following phrases may be helpful to pull yourself out of a shame spiral.

1. I am loved and I matter.

2. I don't need to be perfect to be loved.

3. Sex is an experience, not a performance.

4. This feeling will pass.

5. Intimacy needs vulnerability.

6. Even though I'm feeling _____, I am enough.

7. As I am right now, I am enough.

and sharing personal stories can also be a powerful way to quiet the Shame Wizard.

Rejection

Any way you slice it, rejection stings. There's even evidence that rejection is perceived similarly in the brain to physical pain. The risk of rejection is unfortunately a normal part of the dating process, whether you are dating as a single person, in a couple, or in a polyamorous relationship. Rejection can often be a shame trigger, sending people deep into the archives of their brain and dusting off the paperwork organized under "insecurities."

We often learn to base our self-worth on the approval of others, so if we are turned down in the vulnerable realm of sex and dating, it can feel like we've been sentenced to a lifetime of loneliness. The good news is that the inevitable pain that arises through rejection can make way for profound growth. Dating provides many opportunities to look inward and see where you can practice building a more stable sense of self-worth that is less influenced by the opinions of others. Because, truly, dating is not personal (although, believe me, I *know* it can feel that way); rather, it is a reflection of the space between two people. It is also important to normalize rejection for yourself as a human experience rather than catastrophize about what it means about you as a person or about your future. As you develop your skills of emotional awareness and resilience, you will be better able to weather the turbulent feelings that accompany rejection.

> **Dating is not personal . . . it is a reflection of the space between two people.**

Facing Rejection

This is worth saying again: compatibility in relationships is more about the space between people than it is about the people themselves. When faced with rejection, it is easy to pull out a list of your insecurities as explanations for the other person's disinterest. It is not uncommon while dating to feel that you are being reviewed on your value as a person. And although you may be getting reviewed, it is by a pretty flawed judge. When we date, we always bring with us our family histories, our dating experiences, and our emotional capacity and readiness for a relationship. Attraction is also built on many complex and nuanced factors—they may be irked by your boisterous laugh, you may remind them of an annoying relative, or your impeccable Dwight Schrute impersonation may freak them out—all things that you either cannot change or wouldn't want to because they are a key piece of who you are.

When faced with the discomfort of rejection, people typically respond in a similar way as they do to shame: either by internalizing ("*something is wrong with me*") or externalizing ("*something is wrong with you*"). When taken to the extreme, externalizers respond to rejection with aggression or sexual violence. With both reactions, it is important to remember that someone's romantic interest or disinterest in you is not a reflection of your self-worth. Flirting, dating, and sex are playful explorations of how people fit together—enjoy these interactions for what they are, without expectation or entitlement. Sex and dating are not games you win or lose; they are about genuine connection with other human beings.

Accepting Rejection

A few years ago, I got hit with the age-old "I think we'd be better as friends" by someone I had been on a couple of dates with and was particularly keen on. To soothe my throbbing ego, I took myself out window shopping and was hit with a metaphor that seemed to perfectly capture my experience.

I had wandered into a swimwear shop and started combing through the racks until I came across a one-piece bathing suit that stopped me in my tracks. I was instantly infatuated with its deep violet and coral design with turquoise beading. My mind went from zero to 60 in no time to daydream land, conjuring up images of the vacation photos I would take and the mojitos I would sip in this suit.

I took the swimsuit into the fitting room, stepped into it and hoisted the straps over my shoulders. When I gazed at myself in the mirror, the image looking back at me revealed the least flattering piece of clothing I've ever put on. I looked like I would be right at home if TLC brought back *Toddlers & Tiaras*. Whereas on some days trying on a bathing suit can feel like tests of self-esteem and body image, on this particular day I couldn't help but laugh at how silly it looked and feel relieved I wouldn't feel compelled to spend the money. The bathing suit really just didn't fit. With clothing, not every piece will work for us (dare I mention TLC again here to thank *What Not to Wear* for this

JULIEN CONFRONTS REJECTION

Julien (pronouns: he/him) was an extrovert's extrovert. He thrived when he was meeting new people at parties, networking events, or speaking at conferences to large groups of people. He had been happily married for the past seven years. Recently, he started to notice feelings bubbling up for someone on his recreational basketball team. He brought up his crush early on with his wife, and they talked through both of their feelings for several weeks. His wife eventually agreed with Julien that she would be comfortable beginning a mono/poly relationship.

He began going on dates with his teammate, and one night they decided to have sex for the first time. It was a thrilling experience, which made it all the more surprising when the point guard completely ghosted afterward; she stopped responding to texts and missed two weeks of games. This rejection shot Julien into a shame spiral; he felt like he was a terrible partner and his sexual desires were "too much."

He felt too embarrassed to talk to his wife because he felt he had already asked too much by initiating the opening of their marriage. One day, however, his wife found him tearing up while cooking dinner. She put her hand on his shoulder and his emotions came spilling out. She assured him he was not a selfish partner: in fact, quite the opposite. He had maintained open communication from the beginning and had made sure she was on board before acting on anything. She also told him that his passion and desire to make new connections were some of the qualities that she loved most about him. Julien felt so touched by his wife's empathy and noticed the intensity of the rejection soften. The couple continued to maintain open communication with each other, and after a few weeks Julien was excited to begin using dating apps.

lesson?). This is why we go shopping: to try things on. This is just like sex and dating.

Overcoming Rejection

So, how do you stop rejection from keeping you down? First, give yourself the space to feel whatever is coming up for you: hurt, grief, sadness, disappointment, shame, and whatever else is there are all okay to feel. Opening yourself up to someone you are interested in is vulnerable, and it sucks when they don't reciprocate your feelings. Remember the impermanence of it all, that the uncomfortable feelings won't last forever. Build awareness of your tendency to either blame yourself by internalizing or lash out through externalizing. Breathe, and remember relationships are about fit, not worthiness.

Watch for rumination. Are you stuck trying to figure out where you went wrong? There is a difference between self-reflection and just mentally replaying your perceived mistakes. Although it can be helpful to consider a few pieces of learning to take with you into your next relationship, beating yourself over the head for your blunders like Dobby in *Harry Potter* is a cruel and fruitless form of self-punishment. Remember that the type of person you want to be with will be interested in you even if you were a bit nervous on your first date, had a bad hair day, or laughed so hard that kombucha came out of your nose.

Work on building a mentality of abundance over scarcity. A scarcity mentality can look like a strict belief in finding "the one" or putting people you date on a pedestal. If you catch yourself thinking that the person you are dating is the best and only option out there for you, remind yourself that there are a multitude of people on this planet to be compatible with. If you have a tendency to slip into the scarcity mindset, it can be helpful to date multiple people at once (before you've made any exclusivity commitments, of course) to remind yourself that there are many potential relationship options available to you.

Affirmations for Overcoming Rejection

In the painful moments following a rejection, it is important to show yourself empathy, speaking to yourself as you would a friend, and remember that this difficult moment will pass. If you're hurting, label it as such without needing to explain it. Try out: "This is a moment of pain." It may be helpful to repeat this phrase for a few minutes until the visceral feeling passes. You will not be for everyone, just as not everyone will be for you. The sooner you learn which people aren't a fit for you, the sooner you can collect those who are. Here is a list of tips for dealing with rejection.

1. It's understandable that I'm feeling (_____). I was really excited about that person.

2. Relationships are about fit, not worthiness.

3. This is a human experience.

4. Breathe. Be gentle.

5. There are people that love me for me.

6. I will find my people.

Self-Esteem

With all this discussion around not letting jealousy, shame, or rejection rock your sense of your worth, you may be wondering: What does it mean to feel *enough*? **Self-esteem** is a measure of how someone evaluates their own sense of worthiness. In our culture, we are unfortunately set up to have a volatile sense of self-worth. We are bombarded with messages about how we don't measure up physically, financially, and aesthetically. Happiness, we are told, is within reach if we just buy the barre fitness membership, start using an eye cream before the age of 25, and make partner at the firm. And, if we are not constantly striving for these things, we are considered fat, lazy, or stupid. Because of this relentless pressure, we learn to base our self-esteem on external factors.

Couples therapist and writer Terry Real speaks about three main types of unhealthy self-esteem: performance-based, other-based, and attribute-based. Performance-based esteem is the idea that your self-worth is based on what you can do. This may look like chasing sports trophies, straight As, or promotions at work. The risk with this approach is that you're only as good as your last performance. You can never rest and appreciate what you have accomplished. With other-based esteem, you feel better about yourself as a result of the approval of others. This can manifest through monitoring what you say, wear, or do to please others, or chasing compliments and "likes." It is an unstable strategy because you can't control what other people think of you. Finally, with attribute-based esteem, you feel good about yourself because of what you have: a fancy degree, a big house, or a fit body, for example. Unfortunately, you will be left always needing more and never feel satisfied with what you have.

There is nothing wrong with external validation. It is wonderful to be recognized for things like your beauty, creativity, or hard work. It can get you into trouble when external validation is your only source of self-worth because it offers a brief confidence spike, like a sugar high. It is inherently unstable to survive on the unreliable supply of other people's opinions. Self-esteem based on external validation separates us from our common humanity. It is rooted in comparison—a feeling of being *better than* or *worse than* others.

This volatility in self-esteem can wreak havoc in relationships because we often polarize with our partners: if one person goes to a place of grandiosity, the other drops down into shame. This distance annihilates the possibility for true intimacy and connection. The

BEING A COMPASSIONATE
SEXUAL PARTNER

Sex is about connection. It is not a performance. I wish I could get this on bus ads, milk cartons, and (perhaps, more effectively) condom wrappers. Regardless of what any checkout counter magazine has told you, good sex does not require simultaneous orgasms, 36 mind-blowing oral sex tricks, or a "perfect body." Whether it is a one-night stand or sex with your partner of 25 years, good sex cannot happen without vulnerability, communication, trust, respect, consent, safety, and pleasure.

Just like with polyamory and monogamy, it is incredibly valuable to reflect on what you have been told to want versus what actually works for your body and feels pleasurable. With sex, the more it becomes goal-oriented or attempts to reenact a sexual script, the more your connection to yourself, your body, and your partner is severed.

So, being *good* in bed means having a conversation with your sexual partner about what they are into, as well as expressing your own likes and dislikes. It looks like discussing boundaries and having an understanding of how a limit will be communicated. It is a mutual valuing of each other's pleasure. It is the commitment to doing better than just consent—to not only be listening to words and observing body language, but also aiming to find the other person's "fuck, yes!"

research does not suggest that high self-esteem is a link to strong and healthy relationships, disputing the idea that you've got to love yourself before you can love anyone else (and, yes, I have been warned by my editor that RuPaul is going to come after me on this one!). This can be confusing to consider, because you would think that greater self-acceptance would lead to more satisfying romantic relationships. And it does, but the type of self-love that relates to love for others is based in an unconditional, more interdependent, and stable form of self-acceptance (and the fiber-filled alternative to the confidence sugar high) called self-compassion.

Self-Compassion

In the wake of difficult experiences like jealousy, shame, and rejection, many of us can create more suffering by criticizing ourselves for having these difficult feelings. This can be as simple as saying, "*I shouldn't be feeling this way,*" "*I'm better than this,*" or "*Don't be so weak.*" The thing is, we can't bully ourselves out of difficult feelings. And we certainly can't punish ourselves into being kinder to ourselves. Judging your emotional experiences is just rubbing salt in an open wound. The practice of **self-compassion** is choosing to respond to our moments of suffering with gentleness rather than criticism.

Self-compassion is based on centuries of Buddhist tradition, and over the past decade has been studied scientifically by Dr. Kristin Neff. Self-compassion is the practice of responding to challenging experiences and painful emotions with kindness. It is not self-indulgence, pity, or weakness. In fact, it takes a lot of strength, dedication, and resilience to acknowledge your struggle without judgment.

To practice self-compassion, there are three steps. The first is to mindfully acknowledge your pain as it is right now without amplifying or suppressing it. It can be helpful to use the sentence stem: "Something in me is saying . . ." For example, if you notice the critical thought "I'm unlovable," try rephrasing it to "Something in me is saying that I'm unlovable." This helps your brain understand this is a thought you are having in this moment rather than a concrete label for who you are.

The second step involves seeing your struggles and imperfections as a part of the human condition rather than as a sign that there is something wrong with you. It is the understanding that healthy self-esteem is the equal valuing of yourself and others. For this step,

I practice noticing when I compare myself favorably or unfavorably to others (we all have moments of both). In these moments I imagine breathing myself back to a centered position with others, I inhale imagining sending compassion to myself, and exhale visualizing sending compassion to whomever I compared myself to.

Finally, the third step is literally speaking to yourself more compassionately. It is to use kind and warm language in the face of failure or setbacks. Consider how you would speak to someone you care very much about, and use that same language toward yourself. I appreciate this structure for showing yourself empathy: "It's understandable that I'm feeling (_____) because (_____)."

Self-compassion has numerous positive impacts on mental, physical, and even relational well-being. Neff's research shows that people who are kinder to themselves and more accepting of their own imperfections are better able to extend the same courtesy to their partners. Practicing self-compassion builds emotional resilience through teaching that you are, in fact, able to meet some of your own needs for acceptance and love. Compassion and empathy are not finite; the more you give, the more you are able to receive.

6

Building Stronger Communication Skills

Many of us have learned about tools for developing communication. Perhaps you have heard of using "I statements," active listening, and needs-based communication. Despite widespread familiarity, I have yet to meet someone who is really good at using these tools all the time. Although these strategies can sound simple and even cheesy, they are incredibly difficult to implement in the heat of the moment and with our loved ones. I warn my clients before teaching them communication strategies that they will probably get annoyed with me at some point, because I will repeat myself a lot.

We need the repetition; our brains need the reminders. Like learning a musical instrument, it's a skill that improves only if we practice. Many of us grew up with imperfect models of communication at home—we may have witnessed yelling, name-calling, or suppressing and ignoring conflict. We need to carve new neural pathways to build our ability to tolerate discomfort and distress during difficult conversations. So, although I warn my clients they will likely want to throw the tissue box at me after the fifth time I utter the therapist motto, "And how does this make you *feel*?," when people commit to using more constructive and kind communication strategies, I've seen how it can significantly improve their experiences in their relationships.

Active Listening

To use the techniques of active listening is to be focused and present with the person who is speaking, rather than just hearing the information. It involves making an effort to understand what is being said through full concentration, remembering what is said, and responding in a way that deepens the information. When you actively listen, you hold a nurturing space for someone's communication. Like practicing your musical scales, active listening is a skill that requires practice. It is also the basic skill that makes therapy work. If you've been to therapy, you likely know how different it feels to be actively listened to rather than passively listened to. It can be a wonderful sensation to feel like you can empty out what's on your mind and feel heard. It can significantly lower the feeling of anxiety and distress to have an outlet to feel fully heard.

Being listened to in this way can also you help piece together your existing thoughts and feelings in a way that you may not be able to on your own. One of my favorite images about the process of therapy is a cartoon showing a therapist and a client sitting across from each other. The client's speech is portrayed as a jumbled, multicolored ball of yarn; a few strings of yarn connect to the speech bubble above the therapist's head, and are then being sorted into neat, color-coordinated piles between them.

You don't, of course, have to go to therapy to be heard in this way. If you bring to mind the people in your life that you consider to be great listeners, they likely are busting out some active listening skills. There are tangible tools you can practice to improve your own active listening abilities. These are valuable skills that will help you in your personal and professional relationships. When people in romantic relationships are able to provide this type of support to one another, it can significantly increase the experience of intimacy, connection, and trust.

To actively listen, you avoid arguing, interpreting, assuming, confronting, cheerleading, storytelling, persuading, or redirecting. To use this skill effectively, it is necessary to leave space for the speaker to express themselves fully, as well as to avoid inserting your own opinions, reactions, and needs so that you leave space for the other person to arrive at their own outcome.

1. Shift your attitude to listen to understand, not just to respond.

2. Mirror back what the person is saying to demonstrate your comprehension. You can repeat exact words or paraphrase. It can be helpful to use the sentence stem, "It sounds like you're saying . . . "

3. Ask them to elaborate. You can ask, "What was the best/worst/hardest part?" or "Say more about that."

4. Invite the feelings in. If you notice that the person is talking really loudly or has tears welling up or says they are confused, you can let them know it's okay to slow down and reassure them that whatever feeling they are having is okay.

5. Ask them what they need. Sometimes people can have more clarity on what would be helpful for them after they have had a chance to dump out their feelings. You can ask, "What might make this a little easier/safer/better for you?"

Direct Communication

A common human error we make is to think others are just like us. Because we are only ever directly aware of our own experiences, we can make assumptions without even realizing it. We can assume people have the same needs, fears, values, communication styles, and even personalities. Using direct communication is the best way to avoid making incorrect assumptions. To communicate directly involves taking the time to understand your own emotions, reactions, and desires as well as how to effectively articulate them. It takes courage to state our experiences clearly. Being direct with your language involves trust because it opens up the possibility for the other person to criticize, deny, or ignore

LEARNING TO CONNECT

Aman (pronouns: she/her), currently single and dating, experienced pain anytime she had sex with a partner. She was pain-free, however, when she masturbated. In therapy, I asked her to explain to me what she thought the difference was between her solo and partnered sexual activity. Aman explained that when she was alone, she knew that she could avoid the places on her vulva that hurt and pinpoint the locations that brought her pleasure. When she was with a partner, she noticed that her body was stressed and tense, anticipating the stinging pain that happens when she is touched in a sensitive area. She avoided talking about the pain she experienced with partners out of fear that they would reject her for being too "high maintenance," so she often just tried to push through the pain.

She also longed for sex to be simpler for her and wished she could have the ease of having a spontaneous sexual experience without needing to have a big conversation beforehand. I empathized with her frustration and reflected that accepting her body as it is may involve a grieving of what it is not. I also highlighted that having these types of conversations with sexual partners may very likely mean more satisfying sex for her over the long term. We spent a few sessions exploring her nervousness around describing what felt good in her body and practiced some ways she could open the conversation. She eventually took a risk and explained what felt good to a partner. In our next session Aman told me how relieved she was to see that it was no big deal to her partner, and that this person was super appreciative. Over time, she continued to build more confidence talking about her sexual needs, so much so that it just became a part of her typical sexual experience.

what you've put forward. Direct communication flows in both directions, because it also involves listening with an open-minded curiosity and checking your understanding with the other person.

It's okay if direct communication doesn't come naturally to you; it's often challenging for most of us. The good news is that it is a skill everyone can learn and improve. Here are some tips for communicating directly:

→ Notice your physical and emotional responses.

→ Identify what need is underneath.

→ Use "I statements"; for example: "When ___ happens, I feel ___," "I find it challenging when ___," or "I'd really love it if ___."

→ Remind yourself that everyone has different opinions, needs, and communication styles. Be on the lookout for when you make assumptions.

→ Check your understanding of what the other person is communicating. You can try: "I just want to check my understanding," "I'm wondering if you're needing ___," or "When you said ___, did you mean ___?"

Foster Safety and Honesty through Compassionate Communication

Nonviolent communication (also known as *compassionate communication*) is an approach created by Marshall Rosenberg in the 1960s. It is based on the premise of needs-based communication with others. Since then, a variety of different communication models emerged based on similar principles. I like the model called the "feedback wheel" created by Janet Hurley and adapted by Terry Real because it is a clear and straightforward approach to effective communication. It is a model that I write out for almost all my couples in therapy, and I refer back to it often. It is an approach that can feel a little awkward and overly formal at first, but the more you practice it, the more it will seep into your everyday conversation. In a way, it is like learning a new language.

Some of the key principles of using an approach like nonviolent communication or the feedback wheel are to shift your communication to speak only from your own experience and perspective, to prioritize your care for the relationship, and to ditch the win/lose mentality of communication. You are talking together because you want to make things better, and this often involves compromises and concessions.

Efforts to improve your communication are always beneficial. It is particularly productive in the context of a romantic relationship if all parties are aware of the same communication model and are working together to improve. Within your romantic relationship, before beginning to use the steps of the feedback wheel with your partner, ask them if they are free to talk about something with you. You want to avoid just dumping information onto them if they are already in a mindset where they are rushed, overwhelmed, or need to pay attention to some other needs first. I recently heard the acronym HALT (hungry, angry, lonely, tired) as a self-assessment for if you need to tend to some other needs before engaging in a more focused discussion.

Once you have established that it is a good time to carry out the conversation, the first step is to describe as objectively as possible the event that prompted the need for this discussion. Consider what sounds and images would be captured if a video camera were recording. For example, "When you left the house an hour earlier this morning," rather than "When you abandoned me this morning." A video camera could not establish that you were abandoned.

For step two, share the feeling the event brings up for you. For this step, the simpler, the better. This may also be a great time to break out the "Feelings Wheel" from chapter 5. A common trap people fall into when identifying an emotion is to instead list a thought, a criticism, or an interpretation. If you've ever seen "I statements" misused, this is often where it goes wrong. "I feel that you're a jerk" might be satisfying to say in the moment, but it is not very productive communication. Instead, a more accurate description of a feeling would be "I feel worried/hurt/sad," and so on.

Step three is where you explain what meaning you made of this event. I like the sentence stem, "The story I'm telling myself is . . . " I find this step is particularly beneficial because we are meaning-making creatures. We are constantly taking in information around us and consciously and unconsciously trying to make sense of it. This step is not your opportunity to criticize or lay out all your past gripes. Rather, this is your chance to fact-check the explanation you've created for this incident that is causing you distress. Avoid using the words "always" and "never." When we make sweeping statements like this, it only puts our partners on the defensive to think of exceptions. Step two in this example could look like, "The story I'm telling myself is that you felt the need to get away from me and you want to end our relationship."

The final step is to express a need to your partner. Tell them one thing they could say or do to help invite repair or connection. Our partners can't read our minds. Most of the time our partners want to help us, but they just need some guidance on what they can do. You can say: "One thing that would help me feel a little better is . . . "

Our partners can't read our minds. Most of the time our partners want to help us, but they just need some guidance on what they can do.

Putting this all together, this example looks like: "When you left the house an hour earlier this morning, I felt worried. The story I'm telling myself is that you felt the need to get away from me and you want to end our relationship. What would help me feel a little better is for you to tell me what was going on for you this morning."

Communication during Sex

Talking about sex before and afterward is just as important as communicating while gettin' frisky. For any sensitive sexual topic like fantasies, boundaries, or requests, it's helpful to make space for the conversation before having sex. Vulnerability and emotional sensitivity can be at an all-time high if you are already in the middle of being sexual with each another. Pick a time to chat in a less steamy environment, like at the dinner table, when driving, or while out in nature on a walk.

Come to the conversation with some ideas of what you'd like to share. It's also okay if the conversation about sex doesn't feel sexy. Think of it as a brainstorming session; you're just throwing out some ideas together and finding out what excites each other. Also, remember that we can feel awkward and have productive conversations at the same time. Know that you are doing a brave thing by being vulnerable and talking about your sexual needs, likes, and dislikes.

Before having sex, it is helpful to discuss your fantasies, particular ways you like to be touched, and what sexual vocabulary you and your partner find to be turn-ons and turn-offs. You can talk about what consent looks like for your partner by asking, "How do you communicate if something is a 'no' for you during sex?" This is where understanding the fight-or-flight, freeze, and fawn stress responses is very valuable, because for many people it can be difficult to communicate a "no" verbally. Your partner can tell you if they can use a safe word or, a hand gesture (like "time-out"), or if they know they space out during sex when they're uncomfortable and would like you to check in with them frequently.

During sex, consider how to give positively framed feedback. For example, "I love this, and could you also . . . " Be sure to express verbally or nonverbally when things are feeling good for you, but only when they truly are feeling pleasurable (fake orgasms don't help anyone!). It's okay if you don't know what you want. Sex is play time for grown-ups; just throw out a suggestion and see how it feels. When checking in with your partner, ask them questions, such as, "What would you like me to do to you?," "How can I make this better?," or "Does it feel good when I . . . ?"

Make sure to leave space after sex to discuss what worked, what *really* worked, and what you would like to do differently next time. Not only is it super fun to reminisce on all the sexy fun you had, but it also provides fresh information for when you get it on in the future. You can have these conversations while cuddling in bed, bring it up over a meal the next day, or send a flirty text talking about what really blew your mind last night. Who wouldn't want to get that text?

Expressing Needs

It's okay if it feels daunting to ask for what you need. It is a skill that most of us aren't taught how to do effectively. Thankfully, the more you practice asking, the more comfortable it will become. Using needs-based language is particularly effective if both you and your partner/s are on the same page. You may wish to read the same book, take a workshop together, or go to relationship counseling to hone your skills. The effort is well worth it. It may sound like an oversimplification, but the more you normalize needs-based communication in your relationship/s, the more likely everyone is to get their needs met.

It is up to you to discover how to communicate your internal experiences, and to stay curious to avoid making assumptions about your partner's needs. Remember that the quality of a relationship is not based on your partner's ability to read your mind. Sometimes your partner will be able to guess a need correctly, but that's just a bonus! Instead, a healthy relationship is based on your mutual desire to learn each other's needs and make efforts to fulfill them.

A healthy relationship is based on your mutual desire to learn each other's needs and make efforts to fulfill them.

The first step to being able to communicate your needs is to listen to your own feelings. Your emotions and body sensations are your best tools to help you figure out what you need. Once you have identified your physical response, as well as what your partner could do to help you feel a little better, speak to them directly from the "I" perspective. In other words, rather than pointing the finger at the other person, speak from a place of expressing your own experience and what could be helpful for you. Rather than saying "You never do the dishes," for example, say, "I'm feeling overwhelmed with getting both dinner and my research paper done. Do you have space to help me with the dishes?"

If you are unsure how to understand what your needs are and how to communicate them, I recommend that you first google "list of relationship needs." There are numerous lists available to choose from. From there, to gather inspiration, I recommend you gather 20 to 40 different needs and write them on a piece of paper.

1. While sitting in a quiet place, read each need out loud and pause for a moment after each word.

2. Notice what body sensations and emotions arise after each word.

3. After reading through the list, highlight 10 needs that stood out to you as important.

4. Now see if you can cut it down to four needs. This does not mean that all the other needs aren't important to you. You are just taking a moment to get curious about what shows up for you today.

5. With one need at a time, reflect on an experience where the need was fully met for you. How did it feel emotionally, physical, mentally? Consider the same for a time when this need was not met.

6. Reflect on what possible courses of action you could take to fulfill this need and what possible requests you might want to make to your partner/s.

Understanding Needs

In chapter 3, I referred to the couples therapy staple, *The Five Love Languages*, which is a book that helps you consider what behavior makes people feel loved. The five languages include: acts of service, gifts, words of affirmation, quality time, and physical touch. The central idea of the book is that we all receive love and appreciation in different ways. We also tend to express love to our partners in the way that we would like to receive it. This can often create an unintentional mismatch of partners beaming out love and not feeling loved in return. For example, my partner is an acts of service kind of guy. The most

CHECK YOUR ASSUMPTIONS

One night when I was away for some training, I video called my partner. He wanted to show me something on his computer, so he angled his phone camera to his laptop screen. In the top corner of his screen I noticed what looked like a tiny chat bubble pop-up with an image of a woman in a tight red dress whom I did not recognize.

I felt a pang of insecurity. My mind raced as I wondered who this woman was and why they were chatting. Rather than ask him, I tried to ignore these anxious thoughts. At the time, I was immersed in studying the pitfalls of modern monogamy. I had gathered that being a good partner meant not questioning or prying into the other person's private sexual world. I assumed that asking him any questions about if he was breaking our monogamy agreement risked my getting labeled "the crazy girlfriend."

My attempts to push away my worries were unsuccessful. My distress built, and over lunch I described to my friend Tuck (pronouns: they/them) how embarrassed I felt for being so bothered by this. I outlined my plan to just wait for my anxiety to subside. I expected Tuck to agree with my strategy, but they did not. Instead, they suggested, "What if you asked him about it?"

This blew my mind. I suddenly understood how I could intellectually understand that it is natural to be attracted to other people, yet still find it emotionally challenging when confronted with this reality. Later that night, I talked with my partner and expressed my concerns.

He responded with empathy for my distress, and flipped his phone to show me that what I had seen was a pop-up ad. He encouraged me to ask questions if I ever felt worried like

CONTINUED »

this again. I felt so relieved—and a little silly for experiencing so much unnecessary stress from a pop-up ad. With that said, what I learned was well worth it.

I realized how important it is to check your assumptions, because they are often wrong. I became aware of the difference between throwing out accusations and approaching a situation with gentle curiosity and "I statements" to express how something is impacting me. I learned that one of my relationship needs is to ask for clarity and share my emotions without judgment.

meaningful way for him to show that he cares is to cook an elaborate meal. Because that is not my main love language, I need to make an extra effort to remember that he really appreciates when I remember to do things like pick up the groceries on the way home or tend to the plants.

Nonviolent communication approaches attempt to identify "universal human needs" that all people share. These include needs for self-awareness, authenticity, transparency, belonging, meaning, and safety. Depending on the contexts of our lives, different needs will be more prominent for us at different times. Every need we have is like a destination on a map; there are multiple routes we can take to get to the same end goal. For example, if you have a need for connection, you may choose to ask a romantic partner if they are free to go on a date with you tonight, but if they are busy, you may opt to call your mom. So, in this example, our need is for companionship; it is not a specific need to have a date with our partner tonight. The specific time and place desire for how this need could be met is a request.

Communication Self-Assessment

How are you feeling about your relationship communication skills so far?

→ What emotional experiences are the least comfortable for me to talk about? Do I often avoid sharing my more vulnerable emotions with my partner?

→ How direct am I being in my communication? How can I be more direct?

→ What am I thinking about when listening to someone else? Which active listening skills am I already using? Which would I like to practice?

→ Do I feel most comfortable talking about sex before, during, or after gettin' it on? What is one sexual need I have that I could communicate to my partner?

→ What are some of my relationship needs?

→ How do I know when I have a relationship need that I want to express?

Communication Traps

Poor communication is a trap we all fall into from time to time. Some common ineffective strategies include communicating dishonestly, passively, through dumping, and triangulating.

Many of us have picked up these strategies simply from observing the people around us. Other times, these are strategies we have gravitated toward as a self-protection against the vulnerability of direct communication. Often these strategies can stick with us out of habit, like fingernail biting or skipping breakfast. Part of becoming a more effective communicator is learning to identify your tendencies toward particular communication traps.

Dishonesty and Withholding Information

Honesty is one of the most important pieces of a healthy and ethical relationship. Of course, it is not expected that you have a responsibility to tell your partner/s *everything*, but what matters is that you share information that is helpful for the other person to know and that affects the relationship dynamic. If you were to randomly poll people on whether honesty is important in a relationship, my guess is that 100 percent would say *yes*. It is curious, then, that honesty is a value that is so often compromised in relationships. People frequently withhold information out of fear of hurting the other person or to avoid the discomfort of vulnerability. It can be scary to risk being judged, ridiculed, wrong, or turned down.

Although dishonesty can be tempting as a protective mechanism, it can be relationship poison in the long run. Withholding information can be particularly damaging when it comes to sex. Our sexual desires are powerful. They don't just go away when we suppress them—just look at the low success rate of abstinence-based sex ed. Many clients I see withhold information about sex from their partners, whether they are scared to tell their partner how to bring them more pleasure, have a fantasy they are nervous to share, or have been withholding that the penetrative sex they have been having is actually painful. Our erotic energy is our life force, and when we ignore or banish our sexual needs, we suffer the consequences, whether that's infidelity, resentment toward our partner, or dissociating from our sexuality. I encourage you to listen to what sexual needs and desires bubble up for you, and to discuss the pieces you feel safe about with your partner/s, friends you trust, or a sex therapist.

Passive Communication

The opposite of direct communication is passive communication. Some people don't directly communicate with their partner because they feel like their partner should be able to read their mind, others use it as a strategy to avoid feeling vulnerable, and some are just reenacting the model of communication they learned from their upbringing. Passive communication can include sending hints instead of communicating the message you are trying to get across. This could look like saying "It's fine" with a body posture or tone that indicates you are clearly not fine. Passive communication can also become passive-aggressive if what is said is a covert expression of anger. Some people communicate passively by asking a question instead of directly bringing up the issue. For example, saying, "How often do you think healthy couples have sex?" and thinking *she never wants to have sex with* me, rather than saying, "I'd really love to touch your body tonight."

If you have a partner who often communicates passively, it is helpful to notice when it is happening and stay the course with your practice of direct and compassionate communication. By this I mean: do not respond to passive comments passively. You can draw attention to it with clarifying questions such as, "When you said ____, I'm wondering if you meant ____?" Passive communicators also often look for subtext in others, so your partner might need reassurance occasionally that you mean what you say. In these situations, just confirm with them that there is no hidden meaning in your words and if there is something you would like them to know, you will tell them.

Emotional Dumping

To revisit the advice of Dr. Oz from chapter 5, we want to be mindful of where we pass our (emotional) gas. We all need spaces from time to time to vent our frustrations. We can do this in a way that is productive or in a way that keeps us stuck and leaves the listener emotionally drained. What differentiates healthy venting from emotional dumping is that dumping is like emotional bulldozing: there is a lack of regard

TINA HANDLES BUILDING FRUSTRATION

Tina (pronouns: she/her) was in a polyamorous relationship and had recently gotten an apartment with her two partners, Sasha (pronouns: she/her) and Kim (pronouns: he/him). This would be the first time all three of them would live together and they were all very excited. Sasha and Kim had previously lived together for two years, and Tina felt a bit timid entering into their established relationship dynamic. Tina soon realized that she was more on top of the housework and had higher expectations of cleanliness than her partners. At first, she was okay to pick up the slack and would gather the dirty socks left on the floor, take out the recycling, and clean the dishes left in the sink at the end of the day.

Eventually, she started to become more and more frustrated. It seemed to Tina that the more she did to keep the house clean, the less her partners did. She noticed that she would be grumbling and swearing when she did the laundry. Because Sasha and Kim had lived together for so long before she came into the picture, she felt she didn't have the right to ask for the household tasks to be rearranged. She felt like it was her responsibility to just mold herself into their existing setup. Tina tried a new approach to handle her frustration: she decided to try to outwait her partners and stopped cleaning up after them. As a result, the dishes piled up, the garbage was at risk of overflowing, and the bathroom mirror was freckled with toothpaste.

With each day that passed, Tina felt her resentment building, until one day when Kim came home and kicked his shoes into the corner instead of placing them on the shoe rack. Tina exploded, exclaiming, "What are you doing?!" Kim was startled and then apologetic. Sasha came in from the kitchen and invited the three of them to sit on the couch and have a discussion together. Tina expressed how she was feeling disrespected and taken advantage of. Sasha and Kim said they hadn't realized Tina was feeling burdened and had thought she just enjoyed doing the cleaning. They ended up being able to work together to create a cleaning schedule and encouraged Tina to express her needs in the future.

for the state of the listener, the same issue may be brought up multiple times or a bunch of subjects may be brought up at once, and the speaker often blames others without taking any responsibility. With venting, there is a focus on a particular topic without unnecessary repetition and there is an openness to engage in a dialogue with the listener and hear their perspective.

With your partner/s, it can be beneficial to get in the practice of asking if they have the emotional space to listen to you vent. That way, if they do not have the capacity to listen on a particular day, they can suggest that you speak to someone else or speak at an alternative time. If you find yourself in a situation where you are on the receiving end of someone's emotional dumping, it is a great time to practice setting boundaries and making requests: for example, that the person talk more slowly or quietly or to revisit the conversation at another time.

Triangular Communication

When you communicate through someone else rather than with the people directly involved with a particular issue, you are **triangulating** conflict. It is a topic that is approached frequently in family therapy because it is a common communication style that creates problems. It is a type of communication people should also be particularly wary of in polyamorous relationships. An example of this would be if you were frustrated with your metamour, but rather than bringing it up with them directly, you speak to your partner about it. This can create a skewed view of what the relationship looks like and be an attempt to have someone support your side of a story.

Triangulation can create particularly sticky power dynamics within relationships, especially if kids are involved. It can be confusing and damaging for kids if their parents gossip or complain about their relationships through their children. Triangulation also happens when someone recruits another person to have conversations on their behalf that they should really be having. For example, a mother may ask her child to ask her husband a question that she herself should be asking.

In polyamorous dynamics, just like within families, it is best to handle each relationship individually. Conflict should be addressed directly with the person or people it concerns. If it does not feel possible to have a productive conversation together, I encourage you to consider having the difficult conversation in the presence of a neutral perspective through counseling.

Express Yourself

Learning about healthy communication strategies often sounds straightforward on paper, but it's a lot more difficult to implement in real life. It's understandably challenging because expressing yourself clearly opens you up to the risk of your needs being criticized, turned down, or ignored. A big barrier to communicating is when we fear it will lead to embarrassment or shame. This is one of the reasons it is so hard to talk about sex. Because of the sex-negative culture we live in, many of us are dripping in shame when we consider talking about our own sexuality.

By opening up about your authentic experiences, you are tossing aside your relationship rose-colored glasses to see what is really there. There is a possibility you may find out some hard truths about your relationship—that you may not be as sexually compatible as you hoped or that even when you clearly communicate a need, your partner chooses not to support you with it. But even so, isn't it better to know earlier if this relationship is a good fit for you rather than years and years down the line? In *Daring Greatly*, Brené Brown defines vulnerability as "uncertainty, risk, and emotional exposure" and states that "vulnerability is the birthplace of love, belonging, joy, courage, empathy and creativity." This means we cannot have meaningful connections without the risk of vulnerability. Vulnerability is your ticket to meaningful communication within relationships.

PART III

Thriving as an Ethical Slut

Now that we've covered what makes up ENM and outlined some tools to navigate the relationship style effectively, it's time for us to dig a little deeper. We're going to talk about the hard stuff that impacts our relationships: mental health, sexual health, relationship transitions, breakups, and the inevitable changes life brings.

The goal of this book is to help you *thrive* in your relationships, and without facing the discomfort and challenges in our lives, we're just coasting through, at best. When we resist, avoid, or numb the difficult experiences, or the parts of ourselves we don't like, we are missing out on the juiciness of life. To be in relationships with others is to be constantly confronted with our own humanity.

My hope for you is to love fiercely—while knowing that nothing stays the same. To open yourself up to riding the waves of change and uncertainty—knowing that sometimes the tide will pull you under. To remind yourself that there is never a point where you "arrive," either with yourself or with your relationships. Everything is a practice—self-compassion, presence, vulnerability, *everything*. Our self-understanding and our relationships are in a constant state of flux, making sense and then unraveling, again and again.

Confronting Challenges

We all have a relationship with our own mental health. Mental and sexual health challenges are a normal part of being human. And yet, mental health struggles still carry stigma. I am encouraged to see these topics more widely talked about through education, social media, and awareness campaigns. Mental and sexual health challenges do impact our relationships, and the more we are able to normalize these challenges, the more we can reduce feelings of shame and help people better support themselves and one another.

The discussion of mental health is often left out of mainstream literature on ENM. A lot of the conversation on ENM is written from the assumption that people are in perfect mental health. Difficult emotions like jealousy are presented as something to excavate and replace with more positive feelings, and if that's not possible, it seems to be implied that these people aren't cut out for ENM. There can be a lack of understanding surrounding how past trauma, a dysregulated nervous system, and attachment injuries can significantly impact our experience in relationships. We need to build awareness that ENM can be a valid choice, even if it is more difficult for some people.

Caring for Your Mental Health

It is surprising that in many books and articles about relationships, there is no discussion about mental health. Communication tools and strategies are presented, with advice laid out in clear numerical steps. Have you ever read a relationship advice column and thought, "Um, duh, I know it's better to *not* criticize my partner," and then found yourself calling your partner a goober later that week? Most of us have a basic understanding about what makes a relationship healthy. If that's the case, why is it often so hard to use these strategies? I'd argue this is because it's an incomplete picture to talk about thriving relationships without also talking about mental health. With one in four people affected by a mental disorder at some point in their lives, it is obvious that we can't understand relationships without understanding how our mental well-being affects our thoughts, emotions, and behaviors.

The way we talk about mental health in our culture puts the burden of the hurt and the healing on the individual. A book called the *Diagnostic and Statistical Manual of Mental Disorders (DSM)* is used to diagnose and label people with a disease. The narrative is, *You are sick, you will always be sick, and let's do what we can to manage your symptoms.* The broader systemic violence of white supremacy, colonialism, patriarchy, capitalism, ableism, and compulsory cisnormativity and heteronormativity is ignored. How can we deny the impact of these forces when we see that the highest rates of suicide, mental health challenges, and sexual violence are within the most marginalized groups? Because of our culture's individualistic perspective, mental health diagnoses can often be a requirement to access funding and mental health services. For many, receiving a diagnosis from a physician can be a validating, illuminating, and empowering process, but receiving a diagnosis can also be an isolating, shame-inducing experience, and can sometimes create a self-fulfilling prophecy. If we believe that our diagnoses mean something is *wrong* with us, our experience will be made even more challenging by the compounding effects of shame.

I am not aiming to deny the value of mental health treatment. Modern medicine is a gift, and it's wonderful that we have medication to support us if our brains need help balancing serotonin. There is no difference between taking medication for depression and administering insulin for diabetes. Mental health struggles are not unusual, nor are they a personal failure.

Because the language of diagnoses is limited and focused on symptom management, in my practice I prefer to use a more holistic approach that not only takes into account societal contextual factors, but also considers the person's nervous system as well as their thoughts and emotions. I use an understanding of trauma to help people learn how their nervous system has adapted to try to protect them as a result of past experiences. We aim to turn toward these protective responses with compassion, understanding, and appreciation in order to make space for strategies and responses that are more adaptive to the person's current environment.

Relationship Trauma

I want to credit writer Clementine Morrigan and sex educator Tuck Malloy for first helping me draw the connections to understanding how someone's trauma history can impact their sense of safety and security in polyamorous relationships—that the feeling of intense distress someone can experience in a healthy and loving ENM relationship is more complicated than jealousy alone. The word "trauma" can be a daunting one. Many people consider trauma to be attached only to extreme experiences of natural disaster, war, and sexual assault. Yes, people can come away from those experiences with trauma, but trauma can also result from a wide variety of experiences. Trauma therapists often simplify the definition of trauma as any experience that is too much, too soon, or too fast.

When trauma is experienced in the context of relationships, it is usually more damaging than trauma as a result of factors such as illness or natural disaster. This is because relational trauma impacts our sense of safety, security, and ability to trust those around us. Often, trauma is also a result of a culmination of different experiences rather than one single event. Complex posttraumatic stress disorder (C-PTSD) is a psychological disorder that can develop as a result of prolonged experiences of interpersonal trauma. The violent systems that we live under (e.g., white supremacy, colonialism, patriarchy) also lead to trauma, with the more oppressed groups most affected.

We can experience major, life-altering traumatic experiences, which some therapists refer to as "big T trauma," and we can also experience smaller-scale attachment injuries that are often called "little t trauma." Both experiences are valid and can be helpful to build self-understanding on how they impact your behavior and way of relating to others.

Poly Squared—Polyamory and Polyvagal Theory

Polyvagal theory was created by Stephen Porges in the early '90s and built on Darwin's work examining our body's evolutionary fight-or-flight responses to danger. The term "polyvagal" refers to the numerous branches of the vagus nerve that connect multiple organs such as the heart, stomach, intestines, lungs, and brain. Porges's work provided a deeper understanding of how our social engagement with others also impacts our sense of security and danger.

Because we are social creatures, threats to our relationships are felt as threats to our safety. When we sense that our relationships are threatened, our brains and bodies activate the same systems that would be triggered if we were faced with physical danger, like an angry grizzly bear. From biological and evolutionary perspectives, our protection as a species doesn't come from sharp teeth or excreting poison; it comes from relying on other human beings in our group. We literally need connection to one another to survive. This understanding helps to put in perspective how threats to our sense of connection— whether through a blowout fight, a breakup, or infidelity—can feel so intense. On the other hand, when we feel connected to others, we can shift out of a fearful response. A calming tone of voice, eye contact, or a kind facial expression are all behaviors that can dramatically shift our nervous system into a sense of safety.

Because ENM is an interpersonally demanding approach to relationships, it can be particularly beneficial to have a grasp of polyvagal theory to better understand your own nervous system responses and those of your partner/s. I will keep our discussion fairly surface-level here, but if you'd like to learn more about the science behind it, I encourage you to check out the Resources section at the back of this book (see page 177). In Deb Dana's book *The Polyvagal Theory in Therapy*, she uses the analogy of a ladder to represent our autonomic nervous system (ANS), which is the physiological part of us, outside our awareness, that works to detect threats and maintain our social connections. There are three parts to the ANS, and if we were to place these on the ladder, the top rung is the "safe and social" part of our nervous system, the middle rung is our "fight-or-flight" response, and the bottom rung is our "freeze" response.

Each of these responses has a purpose, but we often have a faulty censor for danger. People who've had past traumatic experiences tend to struggle with correctly identifying levels of threat—either being overly cautious or completely oblivious. **Neuroception** is the term used in polyvagal theory to describe the body's preconscious capacity to detect danger and safety. Shifts in perceived threat in our environment can move our nervous system state from a feeling of calm connection with others to a stress response of fight, flight, or freeze.

Our safe and social mode is where we are relaxed, playful, open-minded, and curious. We are more easily able to be present, be creative, and connect intimately with others in this position. It is most productive to have difficult conversations in your relationship when you are in this state.

If danger is perceived, we will slide down the ladder toward the stress response that the body chooses to offer the best chance of survival in the situation. If it seems possible, it will engage the fight-or-flight response. This can manifest as obviously as clenching your fists and taking a swing or as subtly as criticizing the other person or even yourself. The fight-or-flight response brings with it a whole host of physiological changes, including an increased heart rate and blood rushing to the limbs to take quick action, and we shift into our emotional brain and out of our mental capacity to think more analytically.

Finally, if our body doesn't see it's possible to fight off or avoid the threat, it will drop into the lowest rung on the ladder, the freeze response. In this place the heart rate drops significantly, we withdraw from others, and mentally check out. Sometimes this can look like distracting yourself on your phone or feeling unable to speak or move. Gaps in memory can also be an indication that your body went into a freeze response, which I find to be one of the most amazing strategies our brains use to keep us safe from frightening memories. It is also important to mention that we can also engage in a "fawn" or a "tend and befriend" response. This isn't a nervous system response, but a learned behavior that can be used in times where our brains deem that the safest course of action is not to rock the boat. This can look like people-pleasing or "going with the flow," making every attempt possible to maintain the status quo and stay safe.

Polyvagal Theory in Your Relationship

We all experience shifts in our nervous system throughout the day. Because of our past experiences, we may respond with more stress or fear than the situation warrants. And though often overused, the word "triggered" is a helpful way to understand this type of reaction. We trigger each other in our romantic relationships. All. The. Time.

Let's say you grew up with a mother who texted you frequently while you were out living your sk8r boi dreams. This was irritating because it felt like your mom didn't trust your judgment. Now, in your romantic relationship, when your partner texts you while you are out skateboarding, you notice that you feel a heated frustration. Your reaction feels stronger than the situation warrants. That's because the text was a trigger to your past attachment injury.

The good news is that the more you learn about your own nervous system responses, the more you begin to develop strategies to regulate yourself as well as co-regulate with your partner. It is possible to climb back up the ladder to the "safe and social" zone after sliding down. When we are feeling overwhelmed or shut down, we can self-regulate by grounding ourselves in the present moment (focus on your senses and list smells, sounds, and colors in your environment).

Increasing Self-Awareness with the Polyvagal Ladder

You can increase your self-awareness of your position on the polyvagal ladder and also your personal warning signs for when you're starting to shift to a state of stress or shut down. Take some time to reflect on the following questions. I also encourage you to go through these questions with your partner/s as well. The better you understand each other's nervous system responses, the better you can help support and regulate each other.

1. How do I know I'm in my **safe and social mode**? How does my body feel? What emotions are most present? How would I describe my thinking pattern? What type of behavior do I show?

2. How do I know I'm in my **fight-or-flight mode**? How does my body feel? What emotions are most present? How would I describe my thinking pattern? What type of behavior do I show?

3. How do I know I'm in my **freeze**? How does my body feel? What emotions are most present? How would I describe my thinking pattern? What type of behavior do I show?

4. How can I **regulate** myself and move back to **safe and social** if I'm in a stress response?

5. How can my partner and I **co-regulate** and move back to **safe and social** if one of us is in a stress response?

THE POLYVAGAL LADDER

LADDER	NERVOUS SYSTEM RESPONSE	HOW DO I KNOW?	WHAT I CAN DO	WHAT WE CAN DO
VENTRAL VAGAL	Safe and Social	• I feel safe, relaxed, connected	• Aim to stay	• Aim to stay
SAFE		• I can hold eye contact	• Great place for engaging in creative endeavors	• Good place to have challenging conversations
SOCIAL		• I am curious • I am empathic • I can laugh at myself		
SYMPATHETIC	Fight-or-Flight	• My heart beats faster, my chest gets tight, my breath is shallow	• Pause. Breathe. Acknowledge my nervous system	• A hug • Eye contact • Kind words and affirmations
MOBILIZED		• My thoughts race	• Check in with what my body needs	
FIGHT-OR-FLIGHT		• I am self-critical • I feel panicky • I have a sense of urgency	• Grounding exercises • Nature • Pets • Movement	
DORSAL VAGAL	Freeze	• Zoned out and distracted	• Change my body temperature *(wrap a blanket or splash cold water)*	• Have my partner hold me tight
IMMOBILIZED		• Stiff body posture • Difficulty speaking	• Alternate nostril breathing	• Have partner remind me of a positive memory we have together
COLLAPSED		• Can't make eye contact • Desire to engage in numbing behaviors	• Notice my 5 senses in the moment	• Listen to our favorite song together or watch our favorite cat video

Note: This is just one example of how this table can be filled out and is not an exhaustive list of answers; everyone will fill out these sections differently.

Breathe deeply and ask what your body needs (a snack? a nap? a walk?). To co-regulate with your partner, check in and negotiate what works best for both of you. This could include a hug, sex, sitting close but not touching, goofing around, eye contact, or exchanging kind words. Finally, regulating in a group through connection based on collective rhythm, song, movement, or expression can be a particularly powerful experience. We see examples of this worldwide through practices such as martial arts, chanting, breath work, drumming, dancing, singing, and even spin class.

The table on the previous page shows the different levels of the polyvagal ladder, the corresponding nervous system responses, and examples of how these responses commonly manifest. It also provides notes on how to respond to these states, both as an individual and as a couple. Keep in mind that these are just examples and your individual responses and needs might be different.

Attachment Theory

In simplest terms, **attachment theory** is a system of knowledge originally developed by John Bowlby and Mary Ainsworth that explains how we approach and behave in intimate relationships. Attachment theory is particularly helpful for navigating the multiple dynamics in ethical non-monogamy because it provides insight into your patterns in relationships, as well as those of your partners. The broadest way to sort attachment styles is between secure and insecure attachment. While just over 50 percent of the population exhibits secure attachment styles, the other half exhibits insecure attachment styles, known as anxious or avoidant attachments. It is also possible to exhibit a combination of anxious and avoidant tendencies, which is called "disorganized" or "fearful-avoidant" attachment. Whereas secure, anxious, avoidant, and disorganized are the primary categories of attachment behaviors, attachment style is on a spectrum and there is significant variation within each of these groups.

These attachment styles are thought to develop out of a combination of environmental factors, genetics, and our early experiences with our caregivers. I encourage you to look at your attachment style as you would your astrological sign: not everything will resonate, but the pieces that do may provide illuminating information about your patterns of behavior. In the following section, I will give a brief overview of various attachment styles, but if any of this resonates with you, I encourage you to do a deeper dive into the subject; there are some fantastic resources listed on page 177.

Secure Attachment

People tend to develop a secure attachment style when they were consistently and reliably attuned to by their caregiver as a child. This doesn't mean perfect responsiveness, as this is not possible for any parent or caregiver, but responsive enough. When the child was hungry, they were fed; when they cried, they received support; and if the caregiver missed one of these cues or was distracted, they took time to repair the relationship with the child. This leaves the child feeling confident that their needs will be met and that their caregiver is available for support. As an adult, this behavior typically looks like someone who is able to move toward intimacy at a reasonable pace and is comfortable with closeness, but is also comfortable with distance from their romantic partner. They can comfortably trust their partner, hold firm but flexible boundaries, have tools to self-soothe, and are also able to ask for support when they need it.

Anxious Attachment

The strength of the **anxiously attached** person is their capacity for deep intimacy. Unlike someone with a secure attachment style, however, an anxiously attached person feels distressed when they sense physical or emotional distance from their partner. They worry that they care more about their partner than their partner cares about them, and they carry a sense of not being "good enough" in relationships.

Anxiously attached folks are often people pleasers, constantly aiming to stay away from conflict and keep others happy.

They typically had inconsistent support from a caregiver while growing up, and as a result they become hyper-focused and sensitive to any potential sign of threat in their relationships. The anxiously attached person has trouble understanding why their needs got met sometimes as a child, but not all the time, and as a result they conclude that not only do they need to play the role of *Ace Ventura: Relationship Threat Detective,* but they also need to intensify the expression of their need to ensure it gets met. In childhood, examples can include crying intensely or throwing tantrums in an attempt to meet a need, and if the need is not met, the child experiences severe distress as well as a push to continue seeking connection to their attachment figure. As an adult, this can look like attempts to seek closeness through texting, initiating conversation, or seeking physical intimacy from a place of distress.

If you are someone who is anxiously attached, there are measures you can take to help manage the stress you feel in relationships. First, it is helpful to make efforts to develop your sense of self outside your romantic relationship, whether it is through fostering your connections with friends and (if you are polyamorous) other partners, or pursuing hobbies and interests. This will help you understand how you are not defined by a single relationship. Anxiously attached folks can also benefit from building their tolerance for conflict in relationships and improving their assertiveness and boundary-setting skills. This work can be made a lot easier if your partner is dependable, supportive, and openly communicative.

Avoidant Attachment

In much of the literature on attachment theory, the **avoidant attachment** style is often presented as someone who is cold, distant, and uncaring. In my work with clients who have avoidant tendencies, I have seen this to be frequently proven wrong. Often, people with avoidant qualities care so much that they pull back to protect themselves because they fear getting hurt in relationships.

It is important to remember that, like other insecure attachment styles, people who are avoidant adults also experienced attachment injuries while growing up. Most commonly, they had a caregiver who was either too invasive or neglected their needs. For those who had boundaryless caregivers, intimacy can feel dangerous, as though their identity is at risk of being completely swallowed up and lost in the other person. If someone experienced neglectful caregiving, the person learns to expect that their needs will not be met so as not to be disappointed. With either upbringing, the avoidantly attached person learns to create a protective shell. They come to prioritize independence, and rather than turning to a partner for support, they learn to self-soothe. They also can unconsciously create distance from their partners by focusing on their flaws, fantasizing about "the one that got away," not responding to texts or calls, overly focusing on their career at the expense of their relationships, and sometimes developing an inflated sense of their own self-worth. It is challenging for people with avoidant attachment styles to feel close to someone because they are distrustful that relationships can have both intimacy and healthy boundaries.

If you identify with the avoidant attachment style, it is beneficial to take stock of your unhelpful beliefs about relationships. It is possible that you have been hurt in past relationships, and as a result have pessimistic predictions for relationships. Remind yourself to keep an open mind and that you have the possibility to create joyful and meaningful connections. Know that you can decide how much or how little you would like to open up to someone. Avoidantly attached people often believe vulnerability is an all-or-nothing process and feel pressure to bare their soul before they feel ready. When you are dating someone, you can open up to them in stages while you build trust in the relationship.

Disorganized Attachment

People who have a disorganized attachment style display both anxious and avoidant tendencies. Their early childhood experiences may have been with an attachment figure who was emotionally or physically abusive, intrusive, or highly dysregulated. This environment leaves the child feeling afraid to reach out to their caregiver because they are unsure how they will respond. This puts the child in an impossible situation where they depend on their caregiver for survival, but also want to protect themselves from the caregiver's distressing behavior. As a result of this dilemma, many people who have disorganized attachment styles as adults oscillate between anxious and avoidant attachment behaviors.

Often with the disorganized attachment style, there is a history of serious relational trauma or rejection. If you identify with this category, it is helpful to slowly and compassionately begin to acknowledge the hurt you've experienced. This process is often beneficial to go through with the support of a therapist. Because this attachment style is often born out of a history of serious relational trauma or rejection, it can be very challenging to trust others. The ability to trust others again arises out of the lifelong process of healing your attachment wounds, building your sense of self-worth, and articulating firm but flexible boundaries.

Earning Secure Attachment

Our attachment styles are thought to remain relatively stable throughout our lifespan, but are malleable to change. Prominent experiences of love and heartbreak can also affect our attachment behaviors. It is possible to engage in recovery work through healthy relationships with securely attached partners, therapy, and other forms of personal growth focused on healing and re-parenting yourself.

The attachment literature often strongly suggests that the remedy to the anxiously attached person's distress is to end their relationships if they are with an avoidant partner and search for someone who is securely attached. Although shacking up with a secure partner can be very beneficial for the anxiously attached person, it is often challenging. Anxious and avoidant people tend to be drawn to one another like a moth to a flame. This is because the way they relate to one another unconsciously reinforces their deep-seated beliefs about relationships.

These relationships tend to be characterized by a push-pull dynamic: the anxious person pushes for connection, the avoidant person pulls away, and both people feel unsatisfied but comfortable because this replicates the experience of their childhood. It also creates a sort of "addiction" because when they both land in a rare moment of intimacy together, it can be felt like a "high." Because this feeling occurs so rarely, it can lead to a tireless pursuit of the next "hit," particularly on the part of the anxiously attached person. With all these factors considered, it is possible for the anxious-avoidant pair to work toward a healthy relationship, but it takes the brave and focused work of learning your attachment patterns, understanding your partner's triggers, and developing skills to handle conflict effectively.

Regardless of your attachment style, it is possible to successfully navigate ENM. Although certain pairings, such as the anxious-avoidant match, can require more work, it can also be quite a healing experience to have two individuals make efforts to correct their unhelpful patterns learned in childhood. The key here is that it takes *both* partners being committed to doing the work. If both partners are on board, the journey to earning secure attachment together involves a balance of learning co-regulation skills as well as regulating yourself, prioritizing the love for the relationship over "winning" arguments, developing healthy boundaries, and tuning in to your partner's emotional needs.

Caring for Your Sexual Health

In our erotophobic culture, the risk for STIs is often noted as a reason to steer clear of ethical non-monogamy. Yes, having multiple partners means there are more opportunities to catch an STI, but this risk isn't much higher than other forms of modern-day monogamy. For example, the most common form of relating in our society is *serial monogamy*, in which someone will be with one person at a time. Typically, until someone lands in a monogamous relationship, they will have dated and had sex with a variety of different people. The label of monogamy can often create a false sense of security, leading people in this type of relationship to be less inclined to get sexual health testing and use safer sex measures.

The label of monogamy also does not ensure sexual fidelity. In fact, up to a quarter of married couples admit to cheating on their spouses. What may be shocking to some, and obvious to others, is that the likelihood of contracting HIV and other STIs is actually highest in relationships that are said to be monogamous. The increased risk happens with couples who have unprotected sex with each other, yet someone is having sneaky secret sex. One study in *The Journal of Sexual Medicine* exposed how people who cheat in the context of monogamous relationships are less likely to use safer sex measures than ENM folks. The same study also identified that ENM individuals more frequently discuss sexual health, sexual boundaries, and more regularly get STI testing, and use protection more than the general population.

Sharing Sexual Health Information

Having direct, clear, and honest conversations with your sexual partners about sexual health is key to being a responsible sexual partner. It is understandable if it feels uncomfortable to bring up safer sex practices and sexual histories, but remember: you can feel awkward and have productive conversations at the same time! It is necessary to have these conversations to make sure that everyone involved is making informed decisions. So although it might feel awkward beginning the conversation, once you get going, it often becomes a lot more comfortable.

When initiating the safer sex conversation, remind yourself that this is a normal and valuable topic, and your partner will likely be glad you brought it up. Tell your sexual partner that you care about them and their health. Sharing your own sexual history first will likely help your partner feel more comfortable. If you both are due for testing, you can suggest getting tested together. You can share your sexual history if your testing is up to date, or even suggest that you get tested together.

STI Risk and Prevention

I have appreciated the shift in language in recent years away from "safe sex" to "safer sex" because there are always risks when we have sex,

BREAKING THE ICE

Greg (pronouns: he/him) suddenly found himself single for the first time in three years. He identified as a polyamorous person, and the two relationships he had been involved in recently ended within a few months of each other. Six weeks into singlehood, he learned that he had contracted genital herpes. Now that he was single, the prospect of navigating the safer sex conversation as well as bringing up his diagnosis felt daunting to him.

A few months later, he was a few weeks into dating two different people. He felt lucky that one of his new partners, Tat (pronouns: she/her), initiated sharing her sexual health information early on. She seemingly brought up the conversation with ease and comfort and said to Greg: "I really like you, I want to take things to the next level, and I want to tell you something about myself. I have herpes, so when I have an outbreak there is a possibility you will contract it, too." He felt so relieved to hear this from her that it made sharing his own diagnosis feel like a breeze. They established that they would use condoms for this stage of their relationship.

Greg was very appreciative to have experienced Tat's relaxed and honest approach to the safer sex conversation. This gave him more confidence to approach Zara (pronouns: she/her), the other woman he had been seeing. He expressed his diagnosis similarly to how Tat had. Zara responded kindly, and assured him this wasn't an issue for her because the virus is so common. They both decided that as long as they are seeing other people, they will continue to use condoms and barrier methods. Greg was surprised to learn that having these conversations openly and receiving a sex-positive response also helped erase some of the personal stigmas he had been carrying about STIs.

but there are measures to take to mitigate them. I don't say this as a scare tactic (unlike my high school sex education class, which consisted only of putting up large photos of STIs on the projector), but rather to *normalize* STIs. In fact, when we include HSV and HPV, most people in the United States will experience an STI at some point during their lives. With sex, it is a personal decision to decide what level of risk you want to open yourself up to.

It is your responsibility as an ethical partner to exchange sexual health information if you plan to have oral, vaginal, or anal sex. It is recommended that you get STI testing before having sex with a new partner and if you are in a monogamous relationship, it is best to be tested annually. Barrier methods—like internal (put inside a vagina or anus) or external condoms (fit on a penis), as well as dental dams—are one of the best ways to have safer sex. For further information on the risks, protective measures, and treatment options for STIs, I recommend checking out the Planned Parenthood website and speaking to your doctor.

Navigating Condom Use

When condoms are used correctly, they are fantastic protective measures against bodily fluids that carry the risk of infection as well as pregnancy (98% effective when used correctly). The politics of condom use within an ENM relationship varies. Some people have a strict "always use a condom" policy, and others have more room for flexibility. Although always using condoms is certainly the safest approach to protecting against STIs, there is no one right answer.

The only 100 percent protection against STIs and pregnancy is abstinence, so the decision to have sex involves taking on a certain amount of risk. Everyone has different comfort levels with the amount of risk they are willing to take on. What matters most is open and honest communication between partners about their own boundaries and limits. Honor your sexual partners' decisions by not shaming them for their own comfort level and being fully honest about your own behavior. Consent cannot be present in sexual relationships if one partner is lying about their use of condoms. **Fluid bonding** is a term used to describe couples who decide to have sex without the use of safer sex measures. Some people believe this enhances intimacy in the relationship. Know that if you're practicing ENM and are fluid bonded with one person, or considering bonding with someone new, it is a choice that affects the whole group (i.e., your other sexual partners and their partners), and every person in your circle should be aware of this behavior.

HIV, AIDS, and PrEP

The day-to-day experience of living with HIV and AIDS is dramatically better today than when it was first discovered in the 1980s. If you are living with HIV, you are not alone; in the United States there are around 1.1 million people living with the disease. One in seven people living with HIV are unaware that they have it and could be passing it along without realizing it—which just further emphasizes the importance of getting tested regularly. It is possible for anyone to contract HIV because it is passed through bodily fluids, including breast milk, blood, vaginal fluids, anal mucus, and semen (but notably not saliva).

It can be incredibly distressing to find out you have HIV; often people feel fear, anger, or shame. Taking time to process your feelings with nonjudgmental friends, support groups, and counseling can be really helpful. Although there is no cure, many people with HIV are able to live happy and normal lives by taking a few safety measures.

First, condoms are 98 percent effective against HIV when they are used correctly. Antiretroviral therapy is a treatment that significantly prolongs the person's life and lowers and sometimes even stops the risk of transmission. If someone does not have HIV but is at a high risk for contracting it (e.g., someone in a relationship with an HIV-positive person or an IV drug user), they can take the daily medication PrEP. This pill lowers the chance of contracting HIV by more than 90 percent. For both of these medications, talk to your health care provider to see if they are the right fit for you as well as if you are eligible for programs

WHAT DO I ASK MY DOCTOR?

For many people, talking to a doctor about sexual health can be nerve-wracking. It can be particularly challenging if you fit into a group outside society's expectations of heterosexuality, monogamy, and cisnormativity. Queer, trans, and polyamorous people are often hesitant to speak openly with their health care providers because of the risk of experiencing discrimination. Although in a perfect world, all medical professionals would be nonjudgmental and competently trained in the full spectrum of gender, sexuality, and relationship styles, that is not reality. Often the best way to connect to a sex-positive and LGBTQ+ competent clinic is through word of mouth. It can be helpful to ask for suggestions through online or in-person communities you belong to.

Once you find a doctor you feel comfortable with, it is incredibly beneficial to share openly about your sexual behaviors to help make sure you are getting the right care. To start the conversation, it can be helpful to say something like: "We haven't talked about my sexuality. It is important that you understand my identity and orientation. Is there any particular information you need from me?" It is not your job to be the expert on sexual health testing, but it is important for you to be aware that all people need to be tested for STIs and cancer regularly. Depending which body parts you have, you will need to be familiar with different health measures. For example, a cervix needs a Pap test, testicles require learning how to do a self-exam, and prostates involve regular screening.

to help with the cost. Most insurance plans cover these medications. If you do not have insurance, I've attached a list of state-specific hotlines that help you find a case manager to help you locate funding (see Resources, page 177).

Overcoming Sexual Issues

Your erotic life is so much broader than sex, and sex is so much broader and so much *more* than just penetrative sex. Whereas many queer couples know this to be true, heterosexual partners often get stuck trying to keep up with expectations of traditional sexual scripts. Feminist writer Audre Lorde speaks of how the erotic is a powerful connection to ourselves and our deepest feelings. Esther Perel uses the term "erotic intelligence" to advocate for expanding our definition of eroticism to include its connection to sensuality, joy, and vivacity. The root of many sexual issues is often the anxiety of not measuring up or achieving a particular goal. The expectations that sex should look a certain way—let's say rock-hard dicks, wet pussies, and the enthusiasm of a SoulCycle instructor—and stay that way throughout your entire sexually active life is pretty much a setup for failure.

The majority of us will be impacted by health issues, either personally or within our relationships, that affect our sexual pattern at some point in our lives. This can include anything from mobility changes to hormonal changes, to mental health struggles, to cancer. If you narrowly define what sex is, you are boxing yourself in from all the infinite possibilities of sexual expression. Remember from chapter 2 that sex is a *buffet* of options. To encourage this shift in mindset, many sex therapists are ditching the term "foreplay" because this word means that certain activities have to lead to something else, that they aren't enough on their own, and that there's a natural hierarchy between certain activities, with penetrative sex as the ultimate goal. The truth is: it's *all* sex—kissing, massage, spanking, whatever. Ideally in your life you can have different flavors of sex depending on what you're in the mood for, depending on what works for you in your body at that time. In my sex therapy training, the phrase "pleasure is the measure" was repeated over and over again, to encourage a shifting away from the type of sex people think they "should" be having to the type of sex that is actually worth having. If you are experiencing painful sex or erectile dysfunction, I encourage you to speak with your doctor to rule out medical causes. Otherwise, because many sexual challenges are rooted in trauma and anxiety, strategies such as deep breathing, mindfulness, and working with a sex therapist can be extremely helpful.

Pain Disorders

If you are experiencing painful sex, I encourage you to reach out to your doctor to help rule out physical causes. Often the pain during intercourse isn't just from the physical sensation during sex; it can also be us anticipating the experience of pain. This can happen as a result of having a previous painful sexual encounter, a negative visit to the gynecologist, or birth trauma, or from carrying messaging that sex is shameful or that it will hurt. These experiences can lead the body to brace itself for pain and to tense up. This continues the experience of pain, so the work of a pelvic floor physiotherapists or sex therapist is often to help provide the person with tools to break the pain cycle. Masturbation is also a great way to get in touch with yourself, to notice what feels good and what areas are off-limits at the moment. The better you know your body, the more comfortable and at ease you can be expressing what feels good to your partner so you can relax and enjoy.

Erectile Dysfunction and Arousal Disorders

If you are struggling with erectile dysfunction, I encourage you to visit your doctor to assess for medical causes. The most frequent physical reason for ED is cardiovascular issues. Use of various drugs can often cause ED, such as alcohol, nicotine, caffeine, blood pressure or ulcer medications, antihistamines, cocaine, and amphetamines. A helpful self-check for whether ED is the result of a physical or medical issue is if you get erections in certain situations (while masturbating, in the night, or first thing in the morning), or not at all.

If you never get erections in any situation, there is likely a medical cause for this. It can be upsetting for people to learn that they are unable to get erections as a result of physical limitations. There can be a grieving process involved. It is helpful if you have at least one supportive presence, whether a romantic partner, friend, or counselor. The good news is that it is possible to shift focus from performance-centered to experiential sexual experiences. It is helpful to broaden the idea of what makes a skillful lover, and how it means so much more than having a hard penis. Many people who have ED can find confidence and satisfaction from focusing on giving their partner/s pleasure.

If the cause is more psychologically based, it is helpful to explore where it is possible to create more relaxation and decrease levels of stress in your life. Similar to pain disorders, erection challenges can often be the result fear or anticipation, whether of disappointment, rejection, or feelings of failure. A mindfulness practice as well as speaking to a therapist can be helpful to build your awareness around self-defeating thought patterns. It is also beneficial to build awareness of the pelvic floor muscles (the muscles we use to hold in our pee). It may seem counterintuitive, but learning to relax these muscles can actually help erections by increasing blood flow to the penis.

Orgasm Disorders

Most of the time for vulva-owners, and when medical causes have been ruled out for penis-havers, difficulty with orgasm is a result of stress and anxiety. Typically, sex has become goal-oriented, with orgasm being the measure of success. This mindset leads to trouble because pressure is the enemy of orgasms. If you have fallen into this mindset, come back to focusing on pleasure as the measure for the sexy time that is worth having. Another work I highly recommend for people with vulvas is *Come as You Are* by Emily Nagoski. This book brings me so much joy to recommend to clients because they often tear through it in a week and tell me that it completely blew their minds. It is basically the sex education we all deserve but likely never received. The book delves further into how sexual desire works, relationship dynamics, and orgasms. I love Nagoski's reappraisal of orgasms as "the fantastic bonus."

Lack of or Changes in Sexual Desire

The most common reason people come to sex therapy is for either low sexual desire or a disparity in sexual desire with their partner. People often feel panicked when they notice desire shifts in their relationship. I remind clients that it is completely normal for the sexual energy to ebb and flow throughout the course of a relationship. A relationship will look different 5, 10, 20 years in than it did in the first few months. Interestingly, as sex educator Emily Nagoski summarizes in her Ted Talk "How Couples Can Sustain a Strong Sexual Connection for a Lifetime," the two most important factors in long-term sexual satisfaction in a relationship are that a couple prioritizes sex and has a strong foundation of trust and friendship. To learn more specific strategies on how to build these two pieces in your relationship, I encourage you to check out the References section in this book (see page 185) or seek out a sex therapist.

In ethical non-monogamy, it can be challenging to navigate the dynamics of being at different relationship stages with different partners at the same time. For example, if your long-term partner is in the NRE phase with someone new, it is hard not to compare yourself or feel jealous. At the beginning of the relationship, spontaneous sex often happens more frequently and is usually a really exciting time. There typically isn't much work needed to spice things up because hormones are just doing their thing.

If you're in a long-term relationship, it is okay to look back longingly on the early days in your relationship. But it's also important not to lose sight of what longer-term relationships also provide. Be careful to avoid slipping into comparing your relationship to your partner's NRE. The sneaky narratives of compulsory monogamy can slip into your mind and tell you that your partner's excitement for someone new cancels out the connection you have. This is not true (remember, you can love both Gorgonzola *and* Gruyère). Your relationship is its own entity. Genuine love is trustworthy and flows in abundance. Remember that in your long-term relationship you have an opportunity to deepen a connection with somebody, understand what makes them work, support each other, and feel that deepening of love. Also, the best sex of your life can still happen in a long-term relationship. It can be the chance to learn each other's erotic map and grow together.

8

Growing through Changes

As unsettling a thought as it is, the one thing you can predict with absolute certainty in your relationship is change. You will change and evolve throughout your life, and so will your partner/s. Most of us will have a handful of meaningful relationships in our lives, and some of us will even have them with the same person. This means that the entity that is your relationship is never static. Our relationships need space to expand and contract, ebb and flow. And like the image of the butterfly we talked about in chapter 4, if we hold our hand too tightly around our relationship out of fear that it will fly away, we will crush it.

The price you pay for a deep and loving connection with someone is the risk of pain and grief. For many, this prospect is far too frightening. People fear heartbreak, humiliation, regret, and vulnerability. Frequently, what people fear most of all is actually being happy in a relationship, because this means the stakes for loss are so high that they worry if it were ever to end, they might never recover. To get to true intimacy and connection, you need to sign the waiver where the possibility for hurt and loss is written in the fine print. It is a terrifying and thrilling leap to take into love. It is worth the risk. Sign the damn waiver.

Responding to Relationship Transitions

All our relationships are constantly changing, sometimes subtly like a drizzle of rain, and other times like a sudden unexpected downpour. In my relationship therapy training, I was taught to look at the multitude of dynamics that are in the room: not only do I have a separate relationship with each member of the couple, but there is also my third relationship to the couple as a unit, not to mention the couple's relationship to each other. It's complex! Within all these dynamics, there are a lot of opportunities for change. These layers of relationships also exist outside the therapy room. Not only do we have a relationship to nurture within ourselves, but we also have to devote time and energy to tend to our relationship with our partners. When you start to factor in additional partners through ENM, there's a lot to consider. All those separate relationships (including those with metamours) go through their own ebbs and flows.

Some possible challenging transitions within ENM relationships include your partner starting a new relationship, which can produce the rush of their NRE. This may mean seeing your partner less for a while, which can bring up feelings of longing, loneliness, and jealousy. ENM relationships can also face a changing of hierarchies if a couple uses a primary/secondary model. This can bring up a lot of complicated emotions, even if the change is in the best interests of everyone. If partners have kids, this can also be complicated to navigate. It is not unlike dating as a single parent, where careful thought is put into decisions around when to introduce children to new partners. Poly partners can also have blended families, so any transitions that happen within this context require a lot of sensitivity around the impact on the children.

GROWING THROUGH CHANGE

April (pronouns: she/her) and her husband Noah (pronouns: he/him) were in an open marriage. Because she spent weeks at a time away for work, the couple had decided to open up their relationship to allow sexual connections with others when they were apart. They remained primary partners with each other, and had an expectation that they were monogamous when April was at home. Noah would pursue casual sex with people he met on Tinder. April started out similarly, but ended up hitting it off with a guy named Liam. Their connection progressed to the point where she would stay with him on her work trips.

Noah was in the loop and comfortable with all of this, until April shared the news that Liam was being relocated for work. They would now all be living in the same city, which had not been expected or planned. April asked her husband for a shift in their relationship so she could spend a few nights a week at Liam's place. This thought was very unsettling to Noah, but he felt too embarrassed to share his fears with her. Instead, Noah would make passive-aggressive comments and pick fights with his wife. The energy at home was really tense for a while, until one day they had a big fight over who ate the leftover pizza. After about 15 minutes of arguing, Noah started to laugh, and then cried. He began to open up about his fears and feelings of insecurity. April was able to better understand Noah's perspective and from that point, they were able to open the discussion of what they both needed to accommodate this change in their relationship. With ongoing challenging conversations, they have been able to better navigate the new structure in their relationship that allowed space for processing the difficult feelings and supporting each other.

Your Partner's Partners

There is a lot of variation in how people in ethically non-monogamous relationships approach their partner's partner, or metamour. It varies from no contact to everyone living together as a polycule, to anything and everything in between. Some practice a **kitchen table poly** structure where everyone is comfortable enough with each other's partners that they could sit down at the kitchen table together and hang out before they go on a date with their partner. There is no script for the best way to interact with your metamour; it is something that is co-constructed within the context of your relationship.

The potential expansion of your relationship's support network is one of the biggest benefits of ENM. Having a metamour provides the possibility for teamwork (e.g., around the house, with child care, financially), and lightens the load of responsibility on you to try to meet all your partner's needs. You may even find that you develop a close relationship together, because you already know that you share the common interest of loving the same person.

Certainly, the ideal is to have a positive connection with your metamour that enriches and simplifies your ENM relationship. However, navigating a relationship with your partner's partner/s can often be difficult and present unique challenges. It is often unavoidable to compare yourself to your metamour and think about why your partner chose them. This can bring up complicated feelings, whether they are very similar or very different from you. It is very helpful if you're able to practice noticing when you're dropping into comparisons, and practice the skill of self-compassion we discussed in chapter 5. It is also sometimes valuable to turn to your partner for reassurance of your unique gifts and contribution to the relationship. You also are not typically able to pick your partner's metamour, so there is the very real possibility you just won't get along with each other. If this happens, I encourage you to think about what your relationship needs and boundaries are. For some, having a kitchen table poly relationship is a "need to have," and for others it is a "nice to have."

MEETING THE PARTNERS

Iris (pronouns: they/them) was in an ENM relationship with their partner Porter (pronouns: he/him). They had met Porter's other partner Curt (pronouns: he/him) casually on a variety of occasions, but hadn't had a chance to get to know him on a deeper level. Iris had been struggling with feelings of insecurity and disconnection in their relationship for a few weeks now. Every time they initiated a conversation with Porter about the challenging emotions they were experiencing, they felt he would brush them off and not engage in the conversation. They tried to initiate a few occasions where the three of them would hang out together so that they could have a space to talk about their relationship dynamic and process some of the emotions that were coming up. Unfortunately, whenever Iris approached these conversations, they were made to feel like they were the only one having a difficult time and that they were overreacting.

Eventually they realized that Porter and Curt were not interested in devoting any energy to strengthening the emotional communication and support among the three of them. Iris continued to struggle with feeling like they were "too much" emotionally, and that they were overreacting. After a few months, Iris decided to end the relationship. Six months later, Curt reached out to speak with them over tacos. When they met up, Curt shared that he actually *had* been struggling emotionally when they were both dating Porter. He expressed that he was so overcome with jealousy and fear that he felt if he spoke about it, it would overwhelm him. Iris realized from this experience that, moving forward in ENM relationships, it is important for them to have a close and openly communicative relationship with their metamour. They also realized that they no longer saw their difficult emotions as a problem, but rather as a symptom of an unmet need for a space to process feelings.

Ending a Relationship

Breakups in ENM relationships are unique. In some ways they are easier than monogamous breakups, and in others they are more challenging. They can be easier in that sometimes you will have another romantic partner to lean on if you're going through the end of another relationship. However, this can also bring up complicated feelings—such as guilt, shame, or fear—while processing the loss of one relationship with the remaining partner. If it was a partner you both shared, there is the possibility of deeply empathizing with each other's pain. On the other hand, it can be more challenging because we all grieve in different ways and at different speeds. You may be in the thick of sadness, and your partner may be walled off in denial. Another challenging component of ENM breakups is that there is the cruel possibility of going through multiple breakups at once.

People often feel plagued with the question of how to know when it's the right time to end a relationship. This is often a decision that is more intuitive than it is rational. This is demonstrated perfectly in the beloved sitcom *Friends*, when Ross is forced to choose between his lifelong crush, Rachel, and his current girlfriend, Julie. To make the decision, he writes a list of the pros and cons of being with each woman. Rachel discovers the list, and is understandably hurt when she sees a long list of "cons" under her name, but Julie's only "con" is that she is "not Rachem" (you can blame the misspelling on Chandler, who was acting as scribe). What this exemplifies is that there's so much weight and emotion tied into Rachel's "Rachem"-ness that can't be quantified—no matter how many cons there were under her name, it was clear that, for Ross, all that was outweighed by her simply being her. If you take some time to be still and sit with how you feel about your relationship, your body will often tell you the answer.

The possibility of ending a relationship can often be so overwhelming that people put off thinking about it for as long as possible. They bury themselves in work, mentally check out—or, in the case of ENM, put most of their emotional energy into other relationships. It is important to take time and space to check that you feel clear in your

STAYING CLOSE

Arthur (pronouns: he/him) and Oscar (pronouns: he/him) met at a party and clicked right away. They had the same political beliefs, loved craft beer, and played D&D on weekends. On their first date they connected over the fact that they'd both recently read *Sex at Dawn*. They began talking about ethical non-monogamy, and how on board they were with it intellectually, but that neither had been in an ENM relationship. Arthur spoke about how he also really resonated with the concept of relationship anarchy, because he had never understood the pressure society put on having a singular romantic relationship. Oscar had come to read more about ENM after his last relationship ended. He described how he'd felt controlled and manipulated in the relationship, and later found out that he had been cheated on. He desired ENM because it aligned with his values of honesty, trust, and freedom.

Arthur and Oscar went on to date exclusively. In the first three months of their relationship, they had a passionate and connected sexual relationship. As time went on, however, the heat quickly subsided and their connection began to feel more platonic than romantic. After six months they moved in together and thoroughly enjoyed each other's company. They had blended their friend groups, spent time brewery hopping, and relished their long philosophical talks over dinner. A year into their relationship, they had a tough conversation together about their mutual lack of sexual desire. They realized they both did not want to end their relationship because they worked really well as friends, roommates, and cuddle-buds. Together they revisited their early discussions around ENM and decided to open their relationship to allow sex with others. They continued to communicate well and navigated some roadblocks, but eventually found that this arrangement worked well for them.

decision to end the relationship. At the same time, if you know that this is the end for you, it is unfair to keep your partner in the dark. If you are still struggling to figure out if this relationship is still serving you, I encourage you to reflect on your relationship needs: How well do you feel that they are being met? Do you feel supported in your relationship? We will never find a relationship where all our needs are met all the time but, as Dan Savage would ask: Are the challenges you are facing worth the price of admission for being in the relationship?

Major Life Changes

Making the decision to shift from monogamy to an open relationship or polyamory can create big ripples of change. When existing couples decide to open their relationship, they can often do so in a way that attempts to control and limit the amount of change as much as possible. This is understandable because choosing ENM means confronting a lot of big fears, such as rejection, scarcity, feeling inadequate, and being replaced. Some people attempt to create a sense of stability by creating structure and rules. This can conflict with the basic human need for autonomy and freedom.

All relationships face this completely normal struggle. It is a balancing act between predictability and open-endedness that will go on throughout the course of all relationships. Know that particularly at the beginning of a new ENM relationship, it will likely take some time to find equilibrium between these two forces. And when you do find a temporary balance, at some point life will take over, and you will need to recalibrate once more. The following are some of the ways to anticipate the effects of change with an ENM relationship.

Reproduction

One potentially awkward conversation that is definitely worth having is to discuss both your own and your partner/s' perspectives around pregnancy and having kids. When people make assumptions about their partner's stance, it can lead to a messy situation down the road. The

SAYING GOOD-BYE

Gwen (pronouns: she/her) and Jin (pronouns: he/him) were married and had two sons together. The couple considered each other to be kindred spirits and thoroughly enjoyed each other's company. Their sex was always pretty vanilla, and good enough for the most part. However, 10 years into their marriage, Jin began exploring more kink and BDSM material in porn and realized he had an intense longing to engage in it himself. When he gathered the courage to bring up his interest with his wife, she had a lukewarm response. Over the next two years, they periodically experimented with some light bondage, but it was obvious that it wasn't Gwen's thing.

Their sexual chemistry dwindled, and they reached a place where it was apparent that they were not sexually compatible at this stage of their lives. After many tough conversations, they eventually decided to open their relationship to help each other get their sexual needs met. Jin felt like a part of himself was coming back to life as he began to explore BDSM through play parties and dungeons. Gwen also felt a sense of aliveness return as she found herself falling in love with someone new. Jin and Gwen began to realize that although they still valued their friendship and teamwork as parents, they both wanted to start the next chapter of their lives separately. They decided they would continue to live together for the next year while their youngest son finished high school. Over the next year they had many late-night conversations, arguments, and tears as they grieved the inevitable end of this chapter of their relationship. Although the transition wasn't easy for anyone in the family, Jin and Gwen felt certain they had made the right decision. It took time to navigate how to approach their roles together as friends and co-parents rather than spouses, but eventually they found a groove and were able to be more present to take care of their family because they had learned to take better care of themselves.

decision of whether to have kids is not an issue on which you can compromise, so it's best to know where your partner stands. Part of being ethical in a relationship is being clear about your relationship intentions, whether that is to have casual sex, live child-free, or to have a long-term relationship and raise a family. It is important to be upfront about your relationship goals and not to plan on your partner changing their mind.

Take time to consider each other's position on unplanned pregnancy. Anytime PIV (penis in vagina) sex occurs between a person who ovulates and one who produces semen, there is a possibility for pregnancy. Using a method such as an IUD or birth control pills as well as a condom is a highly effective form of pregnancy prevention (between 91 and 99 percent effective). Even so, all birth control methods have the possibility for failure or human error. It is risky to make assumptions about your partner's stance on unplanned pregnancy. Consider factors like views on abortion, what happens if the pregnancy happens with a primary vs. secondary partner, and if having a child would mean moving in together.

Parenting

If you are a parent, you will not only be considering the impacts of the changes brought by ENM on yourself, but also on your children. The experience of navigating ENM with kids is not unlike that of a divorced parent who is dating, or in a blended family. The life stage your kids are in will make a significant difference to your experience. A young child will need a lot of care, time, and energy in comparison to an older and more self-sufficient teen or young adult.

When you're balancing the responsibilities of parenting, it can be challenging to find scheduled alone time with your partner/s. Often, if someone gets along with their partner's children, a lot of their quality time can be spent as a group. It is also important to the relationship to find time as a couple, even if it's just a sliver compared to what you'd like it to be. If you are shifting into a blended poly family, it is valuable to discuss parenting philosophies and how you'd like to approach co-parenting. This can often be a hot-button issue and can be valuable to discuss with the support of a counselor.

Career Changes

Our work life significantly impacts how we spend our time and energy. Most of us will go through a variety of jobs throughout our lives, and often this will involve significant impacts on our financial status, geographic location, and well-being. Pressure from a high-stress job will impact our mental health, and so will the stress from a loss of income due to job loss. There is also the possibility that you will make the decision to move for the purpose of your career. Moving may bring you closer to a romantic partner or take you farther away. You may make the decision to shift into a long-distance relationship with a partner for a period of time or indefinitely.

Death

The potential of losing a loved one is such a frightening thought that it is almost incomprehensible. Yet, it's an experience most of us have had or will have at some point in our lives. Death and grief are not topics we are very well versed in as a society, probably because many of us find it too painful to even consider. This silence about loss does a great disservice to the grieving because it compounds their loneliness.

Similar to relationship breakups, the loss of a partner can bring up complicated feelings in an ENM relationship. For the person who has experienced the loss, it can be challenging to know how to turn to their other partners (if they have them) for support. The "stages" of grief (denial, anger, bargaining, depression, and acceptance) aren't linear steps, but rather a description of the waves of emotion that will take turns crashing down. Time will heal some of the hurt, but not all of it, and that's okay. I find it helpful to think of grief as luggage: when you first experience the loss, it feels like you're lugging a giant bag filled with bricks, and as time goes on, the bag changes shape, perhaps to a backpack or even a purse, which you still know is there, but you're better able to move through your day. If you are supporting someone through grief, know that there's nothing that can be fixed, but you can offer a listening ear and demonstrate that you are open to talking about it. It is also helpful to offer tangible support, such as help with meals, child care, and housework.

Closing

Our relationships are dynamic and ever-changing. We do not live in a Disney movie with a happy ending. Opening yourself up to relationships means opting in to tending to the growth of this *thing* that you and your partner/s have created together. The relationship is a living entity, and it exists alongside the individual path you and your partner/s have ahead of you. Keeping the relationship organism alive and thriving demands a constant dance of intimacy and longing, interdependence and independence, rupture and repair. There is no relationship agreement you can set that can anticipate and organize your way out of being human. You can't perfect your way out of fucking up.

We have to stop spinning the propaganda that if relationships are hard, it means we're doing it wrong. To be in relationships is to embrace mess. No, it shouldn't *always* be hard, and if it gets to that point, it may mean the relationship has run its course. That's also okay.

Toxic monogamy culture tells us that all relationship endings are failures. This is not so. All relationships have a beginning, middle, and end. In this relationship, did you learn about yourself? Do you know more about the types of relationships that give you energy, and the kinds that drain you? Did you grow? If so, how could that possibly be a failure?

For my ethically non-monogamous folks: you have chosen a courageous path. It takes courage to read society's script on sex and relationships and take out your red pen to write your own version. To go against the grain can mean facing stigma, judgment, barriers, and challenges. It also means that you are living a life in line with your own values without compromise. To listen to your inner knowing of what you need is the definition of freedom. If you have the privilege of safely being able to love who you want to, when you want to, in any way you want to—use it. This frees us all.

Glossary

ace: Also see *asexuality*.

anxious attachment: A pattern of interacting in relationships characterized by a strong need for intimacy and high levels of distress when relationship security is perceived to be threatened.

asexuality: A sexual identity in which a person experiences little to no sexual attraction. Sometimes shortened to *ace*.

attachment styles: Maps for how we interact and behave in intimate relationships.

attachment theory: A system of knowledge originally developed by John Bowlby and Mary Ainsworth that explains how we approach and behave in intimate relationships.

avoidant attachment: A pattern of interacting in relationships characterized by extreme independence and a strong discomfort with intimacy.

biphobia: Negative beliefs, emotions, or actions that discriminate against someone

who is attracted to more than one gender.

bromance: A term of endearment for a platonic relationship between two male-identifying people.

campsite rule: The expectation that you should leave your sexual partner better, or at least as good, physically and emotionally, as you found them. This refers to decisions about contraception, STIs, sense of safety, and well-being. Originally coined by longtime sex advice columnist Dan Savage.

celibacy: To abstain from sex, often for religious, spiritual, or personal reasons.

cisgender: A term used to describe someone who identifies with the gender that corresponds with the sex assigned to them at birth.

compersion: The reverse of jealousy; a feeling of happiness for your partner's happiness.

compulsory monogamy: The idea that in our culture,

monogamy is the unquestioned norm and expectation.

consensual non-monogamy: A relationship style in which partners consent to everyone having the freedom to be involved in more than one sexual or intimate relationship at the same time.

DADT (Don't Ask Don't Tell): A relationship in which no details are shared with partners about their sexual experiences with other people.

demisexual: People who only experience sexual attraction after experiencing a romantic or emotional connection with someone.

enthusiastic consent: A clear, enthusiastic "yes!," which can be taken back at any time and is given without the presence of coercion, force, or intoxication.

envy: A feeling of resentful longing that occurs when people see someone else having something they want.

equity: Within relationships, everyone has the right to ask for what they need and to have the opportunity for that need to be met, even if it is not *equal* to that of the other partners.

erotophobia: The overpowering fear of the harmless sexual expression of ourselves and others.

ethical non-monogamy (ENM): A relationship style in which people are involved in more than one sexual or intimate relationship at the same time. Everyone consents to the arrangement and aims to uphold the value of freedom and goodwill toward all those involved.

ethical slut: The term was originally coined by Easton and Hardy with the publication of their book *The Ethical Slut* in 1997. According to the authors, the term refers to "a person of any gender who has the courage to lead life according to the radical proposition that sex is nice and pleasure is good for you."

fluid bonding: A term used to describe couples who decide to have sex without the use of safer sex measures.

fuckbuddies: A sexual arrangement between friends where there is no intention of turning the connection into a more committed relationship. Often referred to as "friends with benefits."

gray-A: A sexual identity for someone who experiences little to no sexual attraction. They consider themselves to fall somewhere along the spectrum of asexuality. Also referred to as "graysexual," "gray-asexual," or "gray-ace."

hookup culture: A culture that normalizes, encourages, and accepts casual sex without the expectation of a committed relationship or emotional intimacy.

jealousy: A feeling that occurs when people feel something they have is being threatened.

kitchen table poly: A description for a polyamorous relationship in which all partners get along well enough that they could sit around a kitchen table and share a cup of coffee together. This is often used to refer to an amicable relationship with one's metamour.

metamour: In ethically non-monogamous relationships, this refers to someone's partner's partner.

monogamish/new monogamy: A type of monogamous relationship that allows space for other emotional and sexual connections. "Monogamish" was originally coined by longtime sex advice columnist Dan Savage.

mono/poly: A style of relationship in which one partner is monogamous and the other is polyamorous.

neuroception: A term used in polyvagal theory to describe the body's preconscious capacity to detect danger and safety.

new relationship energy (NRE): The beginning phase of a relationship characterized by intense infatuation. People often can't keep their hands off their new partner and think about them obsessively.

open relationship: Non-monogamous formation in which two people who are already in a relationship together agree that they are free to take new partners.

platonic relationship: A strong relationship connection between two people without engaging sexually with one another.

polyamory: A subset of ethical non-monogamy where all parties involved are aware of and consent to the arrangement of being in a relationship with others with the possibility of falling in love.

polycule: A term that is meant to visually represent multiple equal partnerships, by invoking the image of how the particles in a molecule are connected.

polyfidelitous: A polycule that is closed to other relationships separate from the group.

price of admission: Refers to what people are willing to compromise on or give in a relationship in exchange for the positive qualities that their partner brings. Term originally coined by longtime sex advice columnist Dan Savage.

rape culture: The tendency for our culture to normalize male sexual aggression and sexual violence, particularly against women and marginalized groups.

relationship anarchy: The term for an approach that many ENM people take, which means no specific types of relationships are privileged over others and any relationship choice is acceptable.

secondary partner: A type of bond that occurs within hierarchical non-monogamous relationships. This partner typically has less responsibility than the "primary" partner, such as with emotional intimacy, parenting, and financial responsibilities.

self-compassion: A practice of responding to oneself in difficult moments with kindness rather than criticism.

self-esteem: A measure of how someone evaluates their own sense of self-worth.

self-partnered: A positively framed term meaning "to be single." The term was originally coined by Emma Watson.

serial monogamy: The practice of engaging in one monogamous relationship after another.

sex-negative/sex-negativity: The viewpoint that sexual behavior that is not within the context of marriage or for reproductive purposes is dangerous, deviant, or dirty.

sex-positive/sex-positivity: An accepting and nonjudgmental viewpoint about sex in which all consensual sexual behavior with oneself and others is seen as a healthy part of the human experience.

solo/poly: People who are polyamorous, but live alone and keep their finances separate even if they are dating, in a relationship, or married.

swingers: Couples who agree to have sex with other couples.

third: Someone who is entering into an existing relationship with a couple, either just for sex or a relationship.

throuple: A polyamorous relationship in which three people are involved with one another.

transphobia: Negative beliefs, emotions, or actions that discriminate against someone for being trans or not conforming to expected gender roles.

triangular communication: When communication occurs through someone else rather than with the people directly involved with a particular issue.

unethical sluthood: Any action that controls, limits, or disregards the well-being of others. It is important to note that this behavior would also fall into the category of emotional abuse.

Resources

Attachment Theory

Attached: The New Science of Adult Attachment and How It Can Help You Find—and Keep—Love by Amir Levine and Rachel Heller

A straightforward guide to better understanding attachment styles.

Insecure in Love: How Anxious Attachment Can Make You Feel Jealous, Needy, and Worried and What You Can Do About It by Leslie Becker-Phelps

A resource for anxiously attached people in relationships.

Boundaries

Daring Greatly by Brené Brown

A fantastic resource that encourages people to embrace vulnerability and imperfections, and explains how setting boundaries fits into a practice of self-love.

Meghan Talks

meghantalks.com

A great resource for boundary-setting tools. Meghan is a self-advocacy coach who writes, speaks, and works with clients on a variety of topics, including identifying values and setting boundaries. Keep your eyes peeled for her boundary workbook, which she updates and releases each year.

Terri Cole

terricole.com/setting-personal-emotional-boundaries

A therapist who creates a variety of resources to help people develop their personal and emotional boundaries.

HIV/AIDS

The Centers for Disease Control and Prevention's (CDC) hotline can help you find a doctor near you who specializes in treating HIV: 1-800-CDC-INFO (1-800-232-4636)

State HIV/AIDS Hotlines

hab.hrsa.gov/get-care/state-hivaids-hotlines

thebody.com

Educational and supportive resources on the topic of HIV.

LGBTQ+ Resources and Culture

asexuality.org

Resources and support on the topic of asexuality.

It Gets Better

itgetsbetter.org

A nonprofit organization that supports, empowers, and connects LGBTQ+ youth worldwide.

pflag.org and out.com

Resources for parents and friends of LGBTQ+ people.

The Transgender Training Institute (TTI)

transgendertraininginstitute.com

World Professional Association for Transgender Health

wpath.org

Resources for transgender people and individuals who would like to learn more and increase competency in transgender issues.

Mental Health

The Gifts of Imperfection by Brené Brown

Learn how to embrace your imperfections and move toward a more wholehearted life.

Self-Compassion by Kristin Neff

Written by the leading researcher in the field of self-compassion, this is a guide to navigating the practice of being kinder to yourself.

Polyamory/ENM

The Ethical Slut by Dossie Easton and Janet Hardy

A wonderful entry point for understanding the basics of non-monogamy.

Love Uncommon

loveuncommon.com

A site run by Sophia Graham, a sex-positive, gender-affirming, LGBTQ+ educator and coach. Her blog has a variety of helpful polyamory resources.

Monogamy Detox

monogamydetox.com

A course on the topic of "monogamy detox."

Opening Up: A Guide to Creating and Sustaining Open Relationships by Tristan Taormino

A thorough and practical guide to understanding and navigating different forms of open relationships.

Poly Living

polyliving.net

This site, which includes articles, a forum, and social media, has served the ethical non-monogamy community for more than two decades.

Polyamory Starter Kit

polyamorystarterkit.com

Education for individuals, couples, and therapists on polyamory. They have particularly great worksheets and training for therapists on how to work with ENM clients.

Sex at Dawn: How We Mate, Why We Stray, and What It Means for Modern Relationships by Christopher Ryan and Cacilda Jethá

A now classic book examining the roots of monogamy from an anthropological, archaeologic, primatologic, anatomical, and psychosexual perspective.

Sexplanations with Dr. Lindsey Doe on YouTube

youtube.com/watch?v=0VKGRrOzMDg

A positively framed quick introductory video about polyamory. A great resource if you want someone in your life to learn about polyamory.

Solo Poly

solopoly.net

Blog written by Amy Gahran, author of *Stepping Off the Relationship Escalator: Uncommon Love and Life*, addressing a variety of topics within the realm of polyamory.

Tuck Malloy

tuckmalloyeducation.com

Tuck is a fantastic sex educator who offers classes on a variety of topics, including a course on "Navigating Communication and Relationship Trauma in Ethical Non-Monogamy."

You Can't Own the Fucking Stars by Clementine Morrigan

I can't recommend this zine enough for people who struggle with anxiety, relationship trauma, and stress in polyamory. I have heard from many clients that this is the first piece of writing they felt actually captured their experience in polyamory.

Sex

Come as You Are: The Surprising New Science That Will Transform Your Sex Life by Emily Nagoski

The book I recommend most frequently in my sex therapy work. It focuses on vulva-havers and covers valuable topics related to sexuality and sexual functioning.

Mating in Captivity by Esther Perel

Examines the paradox in contemporary relationships surrounding the need for both secure love and passion.

MoJo Upgrade

mojoupgrade.com

An online quiz you can take with your sexual partner. It presents you with a list of sexual activities you can say "yes," "no," or "maybe" to.

Not Always in the Mood: The New Science of Men, Sex, and Relationships by Sarah Hunter Murray

A helpful book on the topic of sexual desire disparities in relationships.

Sexual Healing: The Completest Guide to Overcoming Common Sexual Problems by Barbara Keesling

A great resource for therapists and clients in working with sexual issues.

Tongue Tied: Untangling Communication in Sex, Kink, and Relationships by Stella Harris

A helpful guide to improve talking about sex.

Social Justice in Sexuality

Ante Up!

anteuppd.com/buy-curriculum

Curricula by Bianca Laureano provide a variety of course offerings, including topics of sexual and reproductive justice focused on communities of color.

The Body Is Not an Apology: The Power of Radical Self-Love by Sonya Renee Taylor

Examines the oppressive systems that impair people's relationships to their bodies and speaks to the power of reconnecting the mind and body through radical self-love.

Pleasure Activism: The Politics of Feeling Good by adrienne maree brown

A collection of essays examining the politics of healing and making social justice a pleasurable experience. A wonderful book for people looking to understand how pleasure is a political act, particularly for marginalized bodies.

STIs

Planned Parenthood

plannedparenthood.org

Numerous resources for reproductive health care.

Positive Results

positiveresults.support/blog

Created by sex educator Rae Higgins, who focuses on providing information and tools to slay stigma surrounding STIs.

Trauma

The Body Keeps the Score by Bessel van der Kolk

An accessible and thorough book addressing the impacts and treatment for trauma written by one of the world's leading experts in the field.

Healing Sex: A Mind-Body Approach to Healing Sexual Trauma by Staci Haines

A resource for sexual assault survivors looking to heal their relationship to their sexuality.

I Hope We Choose Love: A Trans Girl's Notes from the End of the World by Kai Cheng Thom

This can be an empowering book for people (and particularly survivors of sexual violence) to examine topics of trauma, abuse, activism, transphobia, and racism under a transformative justice lens, and to feel inspired to imagine a new and healthier way to move forward in the world.

The Polyvagal Theory in Therapy: Engaging the Rhythm of Regulation by Deb Dana

Further information on polyvagal theory written for both clients and therapists.

RAINN

rainn.org

The Rape, Abuse & Incest National Network (RAINN) is the largest American nonprofit anti–sexual assault organization. There are a variety of resources to support sexual assault survivors.

Resilience

ourresilience.org/programs-services

Survivors can get an immediate, one-time virtual crisis session with a resilience Chicago therapist by filling out a form.

References

1: Recognizing Your Relationship Values

American Psychological Association. Accessed April 23, 2020. apa.org /topics/divorce.

Ballard, Jamie. "Millennials Are Less Likely to Want a Monogamous Relationship." YouGov, January 31, 2020. today.yougov.com /topics/relationships/articles-reports/2020/01/31/millennials -monogamy-poly-poll-survey-data.

Constantine, Larry L., and Joan M. Constantine. *Group Marriage: A Study of Contemporary Multilateral Marriage.* New York: Collier Books, 1974.

Dionne, Evette. "'She's Gotta Have It' Butchers Polyamory and Queerness." Bitch Media. Accessed April 23, 2020. bitchmedia.org /article/shes-gotta-have-it-review.

Emens, Elizabeth F. "Monogamy's Law: Compulsory Monogamy and Polyamorous Existence." *SSRN Electronic Journal*, 2004. doi.org /10.2139/ssrn.506242.

Gahran, Amy. *Stepping Off the Relationship Escalator: Uncommon Love and Life.* Boulder, CO: Off the Escalator Enterprises, LLC, 2017.

Hamilton, Jolene Emily. "Triangular Trouble: A Phenomenological Exploration of Jealousy's Archetypal Nature in Polyamorous Individuals." PhD diss., Pacifica Graduate Institute, 2020.

Hardy, Janet W., and Easton Dossie. *The Ethical Slut: A Practical Guide to Polyamory, Open Relationships, and Other Freedoms in Sex and Love.* New York: Random House, 2017.

Haupert, M. L., Amanda N. Gesselman, Amy C. Moors, Helen E. Fisher, and Justin R. Garcia. "Prevalence of Experiences with Consensual Nonmonogamous Relationships: Findings from Two National Samples of Single Americans." *Journal of Sex & Marital Therapy* 43, no. 5 (2016): 424–40. doi.org/10.1080/0092623x.2016.1178675.

Lees, Paris, Radhika Seth, and Alice Cary. "From the Archive: Emma Watson on Being Happily 'Self-Partnered' At 30." *British Vogue*,

April 15, 2020. vogue.co.uk/news/article/emma-watson-on-fame
-activism-little-women.

MacDonald, A. "Polyamory" enters the Oxford English Dictionary, and
tracking the word's origins [Web log comment]. January 6, 2007.
Retrieved from polyinthemedia.blogspot.com/2007/01/polyamory
-enters-oxford-english.html.

Morrigan, Clementine. *Love without Emergency*. Accessed April 23,
2020. clementinemorrigan.com/product/love-without-emergency.

O'Neill, Nena, and George O'Neill. *Open Marriage: A New Life Style for
Couples*. New York: M. Evans, 1984.

Perel, Esther. *The State of Affairs: Rethinking Infidelity*. London:
Yellow Kite, 2019.

Raphael, Rina. "Why Doesn't Anyone Want to Live in This Perfect
Place?" *The New York Times*, August 24, 2019. nytimes.com
/2019/08/24/style/womyns-land-movement-lesbian
-communities.html.

Ryan, Christopher, and Cacilda Jethá. *Sex at Dawn: The Prehistoric
Origins of Modern Sexuality*. Brunswick, Victoria: Scribe, 2018.

Savage, Dan. "Savage Love Web Extra." The Stranger. Accessed April 23,
2020. thestranger.com/seattle/Content?oid=572102.

"Slut." Merriam-Webster. Accessed April 23, 2020. merriam-webster
.com/dictionary/slut.

Taormino, Tristan. *Opening Up: A Guide to Creating and Sustaining
Open Relationships*. San Francisco, CA: Cleis, 2007.

2: Loving Your Relationship with Sex

Allyn, David. *Make Love, Not War: The Sexual Revolution: An Unfettered
History*. London: Routledge, 2016.

AMS Sexual Assault Support Centre. Accessed April 24, 2020.
amssasc.ca/statistics.

Brennan, S., and A. Taylor-Butts. *Canadian Centre for Justice Statistics
Profile Series: Sexual Assault in Canada 2004 and 2007*. 2008.
Retrieved from Statistics Canada website. www.publicsafety.gc.ca/
cnt/rsrcs/lbrr/ctlg/dtls-en.aspx?d=PS&i=79590011.

Chicago Tribune. "#MeToo: A Timeline of Events." *Chicago Tribune*, March 11, 2020. chicagotribune.com/lifestyles/ct-me-too-timeline -20171208-htmlstory.html.

Davidson, Erin. "What I Needed to Hear after My Sexual Assault." *Medium*, November 19, 2018. medium.com/@erineileen_12198 /what-i-needed-to-hear-after-my-sexual-assault-f9afc6e158eb.

Davidson, Erin Eileen. "#Metoo: Stories of Sexual Assault Survivors on Campus." Electronic Theses and Dissertations (ETDs) 2008+. T, University of British Columbia. doi:dx.doi.org/10.14288 /1.0377180.

"Defining Sexual Health." World Health Organization, January 2002. who .int/reproductivehealth/topics/gender_rights/defining_sexual _health.pdf?ua=1.

Dischiavo, Rosalyn. *The Deep Yes: The Lost Art of True Receiving*. Spanda Press, 2016.

Donaghue, Chris. *Sex Outside the Lines: Authentic Sexuality in a Sexually Dysfunctional Culture*. Dallas: BenBella Books, 2015.

Herbenick, Debby, Tsung-Chieh (Jane) Fu, Jennifer Arter, Stephanie A. Sanders, and Brian Dodge. "Women's Experiences with Genital Touching, Sexual Pleasure, and Orgasm: Results from a U.S. Probability Sample of Women Ages 18 to 94." *Journal of Sex & Marital Therapy* 44, no. 2 (September 2017): 201–12. doi.org/10.1080 /0092623x.2017.1346530.

Ince, John. *The Politics of Lust*. Amherst, NY: Prometheus Books, 2005.

Park, Andrea. "#MeToo Reaches 85 Countries with 1.7M Tweets." CBS News. CBS Interactive, December 6, 2017. cbsnews .com/news/metoo-reaches-85-countries-with-1-7-million-tweets.

Rotenberg, Cristine. "Police-Reported Sexual Assaults in Canada, 2009 to 2014: A Statistical Profile." Statistics Canada: Canada's national statistical agency/Statistique Canada: Organisme statistique national du Canada. Government of Canada, Statistics Canada, October 3, 2017. www150.statcan.gc.ca/n1/pub /85-002-x/2017001/article/54866-eng.htm.

"Sex." Merriam-Webster. Accessed April 24, 2020. merriam-webster.com /dictionary/sex.

"Sexual Assault and Vulnerable Populations." Stop Violence Against
  Women. The Advocates for Human Rights, 2006. stopvaw.org
  /sexual_assault_and_vulnerable_populations.
Statistics About Sexual Violence. National Sexual Violence Resource
  Center, 2015. nsvrc.org/sites/default/files/publications_nsvrc
  _factsheet_media-packet_statistics-about-sexual-violence
  _0.pdf.
"The Body Is Not An Apology." Accessed April 24, 2020.
  thebodyisnotanapology.com.
"*TIME* Person of the Year 2017: The Silence Breakers." *Time*. Accessed
  April 24, 2020. time.com/time-person-of-the-year-2017-silence
  -breakers.
Van der Kolk, Bessel. *The Body Keeps the Score: Mind, Brain and Body
  in the Transformation of Trauma*. London: Penguin Books, 2015.

3: Honoring Your Needs and Fears

Gottman, John M. *The Science of Trust: Emotional Attunement for
  Couples*. New York: W. W. Norton & Company, 2011 (p. 254).
Perel, Esther. *Mating in Captivity: Unlocking Erotic Intelligence*. London:
  Hodder, 2007.

5: Recognizing Jealousy and Other Hard Feelings

Anas, Brittany. "This 'Feelings Wheel' Will Help You Better Describe Your
  Emotions." Simplemost, April 14, 2017. simplemost.com/feeling
  -wheel-will-help-better-describe-emotions.
"Clementine Morrigan." Accessed June 11, 2020. clementinemorrigan
  .com/category/workshops.
"Compassion." Kristin Neff. Accessed June 24, 2020. self-compassion.org.
Hart, Sybil L., and Maria Legerstee. *Handbook of Jealousy: Theory,
  Research, and Multidisciplinary Approaches*. John Wiley & Sons, 2013.
Real, Terrence. *The New Rules of Marriage: What You Need to Know to
  Make Love Work*. Random House Digital, Inc., 2008.

"Your Questions Answered!" Oprah.com. Accessed June 11, 2020. oprah.com/health/your-questions-answered/all.

6: Building Stronger Communication Skills

Brown, Brené. *Daring Greatly: How the Courage to Be Vulnerable Transforms the Way We Live, Love, Parent, and Lead.* Penguin Random House Audio Publishing Group, 2017.

Real, Terrence. *The New Rules of Marriage: What You Need to Know to Make Love Work.* New York: Ballantine Books, 2008.

7: Confronting Challenges

Advanced Solutions International, Inc. "Infidelity." Accessed June 24, 2020. aamft.org/Consumer_Updates/Infidelity.aspx.

"Biobehavioral Responses to Stress in Females: Tend-and-Befriend, Not Fight-or-Flight." *Foundations in Social Neuroscience,* 2002. doi.org /10.7551/mitpress/3077.003.0048.

Conley, Terri D., Amy C. Moors, Ali Ziegler, and Constantina Karathanasis. "Unfaithful Individuals Are Less Likely to Practice Safer Sex Than Openly Nonmonogamous Individuals." *The Journal of Sexual Medicine* 9, no. 6 (2012): 1559–65. doi.org/10.1111/j.1743-6109.2012 .02712.x.

Keesling, Barbara. *Sexual Healing: The Completest Guide to Overcoming Common Sexual Problems.* Alameda, CA: Hunter House, 2006.

Kolk, Bessel A. van der. "The Body Keeps the Score: Memory and the Evolving Psychobiology of Posttraumatic Stress." *Harvard Review of Psychiatry* 1, no. 5 (1994): 253–65. doi.org/10.3109 /10673229409017088.

Levine, Amir, and Rachel Heller. *Attached: The New Science of Adult Attachment and How It Can Help You Find—and Keep—Love.* Tarcherperigee, 2012.

Lorde, Audre. "The Uses of the Erotic: The Erotic as Power." In Henry Abelove, Michèle Aina Barale, and David M. Halperin, eds. *The Lesbian and Gay Studies Reader.* New York: Routledge, 1993.

"Mental Disorders Affect One in Four People." World Health Organization, July 29, 2013. who.int/whr/2001/media_centre/press_release/en.

Perel, Esther. *Mating in Captivity: Unlocking Erotic Intelligence*. New York: Harper, 2007.

Planned Parenthood. "Frequently Asked Questions about STI Testing." Accessed June 24, 2020. plannedparenthood.org/planned-parenthood-st-louis-region-southwest-missouri/blog/frequently-asked-questions-about-sti-testing.

Pleasure Centered Sex Education. Accessed June 24, 2020. tuckmalloyeducation.com.

"Public Knowledge and Attitudes About Sexually Transmitted Infections: KFF Polling and Policy Insights." *KFF*, February 19, 2020. kff.org/womens-health-policy/issue-brief/public-knowledge-and-attitudes-about-sexually-transmitted-infections.

Richards, Christina, and Meg Barker. *Sexuality & Gender for Mental Health Professionals: A Practical Guide*. Sage, 2013.

"Suicide." World Health Organization. Accessed June 24, 2020. who.int/news-room/fact-sheets/detail/suicide.

Trojan Sexual Health Report Card. Accessed June 24, 2020. factsaboutcondoms.com/report.php.

"Victims of Sexual Violence: Statistics." RAINN. Accessed June 24, 2020. rainn.org/statistics/victims-sexual-violence.

Walker, Pete. *Complex PTSD: From Surviving to Thriving: A Guide and Map for Recovering from Childhood Trauma*. Lafayette, CA: Azure Coyote, 2013.

8: Growing through Changes

Planned Parenthood. "Birth Control Methods & Options: Types of Birth Control." Accessed June 24, 2020. plannedparenthood.org/learn/birth-control.

Index

A

Abuse, 8–9. *See also* Sexual
  assault and trauma
Active listening, 114–115
Agreements, 78–82
AIDS, 152–153
Ainsworth, 143
Alone, being, 58. *See also* Singlehood
Anonymity, 81–82
Anxious attachment, 55, 144–145
Arousal disorders, 155–156
Asexuality, 16
Assumptions, 123–124
Attachment theory, 52, 55, 57, 143–148
Avoidant attachment, 55, 57, 145–146

B

BDSM, 18
Biphobia, 23
Body Is Not an Apology, The (Taylor), 37
Body Keeps the Score, The
  (van der Kolk), 43
Boundaries, 10, 20, 38–39, 69–70, 76–78
Bowlby, John, 143
Breakups, 57–58, 164, 166–167
Bromances, 17
brown, adrienne maree, 37–38
Brown, Brené, 131
Burke, Tarana, 38

C

Campsite rule, 6
Career changes, 169
Casual relationships, 18
Celibacy, 16
Chapman, Gary, 50
Cheating, 9–10, 20, 149
Come as You Are (Nagoski), 156
Communication
  active listening, 114–115

compassionate, 117–119, 124
direct, 115–117
enthusiastic consent, 41
of needs, 50–51, 121–124
nonviolent, 117–119, 124
passive, 127
self-assessment, 125
during sex, 119–120
traps, 125–130
triangular, 129–130
verbal vs. nonverbal consent, 39–40
Compersion, 21
Complex posttraumatic stress
  disorder (C-PTSD), 137–138
Condom use, 151–152
Conflict resolution, 82–84, 129–130
Consensual non-monogamy, 12. *See
  also* Ethical non-monogamy (ENM)
Consent, 38–41, 151–152
Constantine, Joan and Larry, 22

D

Dana, Deb, 139
Daring Greatly (Brown), 131
Dating, 85–86. *See also* Rejection
Death, 57–58, 169
DeLarverie, Stormé, 36
Demisexuality, 16
Desire, changes in, 156–157
Discomfort, 58–59
Discrimination, 23–24
Dishonesty, 126
Disorganized attachment, 146–147
Distress, 93
Don't Ask Don't Tell (DADT)
  situations, 69, 81–82

E

Easton, Dossie, 4, 5, 23
Emotional dumping, 127, 129
Emotional resilience, 53, 92
Envy, 92–93
Equality, 52

Acknowledgments

I am so appreciative of all the support that I received through the writing process. I am thankful to Callisto Media for the opportunity to write my first book and to my editor, Brian Sweeting, whose use of emojis in Track Changes made the revision process significantly more fun. To my partner, Shane, who had an unending supply of supportive words, hugs, and snacks. My friends Whitney, Jenna, Liz, Rebecca, Olivia, and Meghan for the encouraging texts, phone calls, flowers, and writing playlists. My family, for always supporting my studies, even if we don't talk about it at the dinner table. My own therapist, Diana Kollar, who has been there with me through some big life transitions and who first introduced me to many of the theories I reference in this book. To the many sex educators and therapists I have learned from and particularly: Kristen C. Dew (LMFT), Joli Hamilton (PhD, CSE), Ann C. Wallace, and Tuck Malloy, who generously gave their time to be interviewed for this project.

About the Author

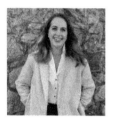 **Erin Davidson** (pronouns: she/her), RCC, MA, is a writer and Registered Clinical Counselor specializing in sex therapy and relationship counseling. She works with clients of all genders, sexual orientations, and relationship dynamics to bring more compassion and joy to their connection with their sexuality, their relationships, and themselves. This is her first book. You can read more of her writing and connect with her on Instagram @ erin.e.davidson and on her website, erinedavidson.com.